HCG Awesome

Success Secrets Revealed
Compiled by Lisa B Ellison

* Everything you need to lose weight most efficiently and affordable is in this book, the doctor's manuscript, step-by-step instructions and over 100 recipes
* Without hCG, the body stores and HOLDS ONTO fat, to prepare for survival during a possible future famine/starvation
 * Without hCG, it can seem impossible to lose weight, as the body stubbornly refuses to release it, and instead s-l-o-w-s the metabolism d-o-w-n
 * When hCG is combined with Dr. Simeon's specific low-calorie protocol, the body responds by RELEASING that stored excess fat
* Your body feeds off of thousands of fat calories per day, so you are NOT starving, and you ARE comfortable and energized
 * Clients using hCG lose weight fast - an average of 1/2 - 1 1/2 lbs - per day!
* Exercise is not required, although you may continue light-moderate exercise, if desired

Table of Contents

My Testimonial

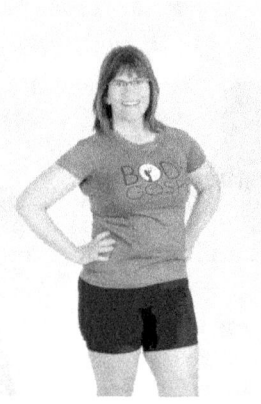

I'm not much of a dieter. I never wanted to count calories or points. So with each kid I got a little heavier and heavier. I have 4 children as with the birth of each child my weight went up a bit. My youngest is now 4. I know you're wondering, so I'll tell you. I weighed about 230, maybe 240, for almost 12 years. I had been tracking my weight online using a ticker for 3 years and spent over two years just watching my weight and it was basically the same weight. Just "watching my weight" wasn't helping.

I thank God for showing the way out of my overweight-ness! I first heard about the hCG diet in a message board where the opinions were polar opposites --- the ones who have lost with it and the ones saying how bad it is for you to go on a starvation diet. In November 2009, I discovered a website named hcgmiracle that was quite new. I ordered the homeopathic drops and started on Thanksgiving. 23 days lost 20 lbs. I'm glad I ordered the drops through them because they have great support and have online classes telling me what to eat, etc. step by step. I paid over $100 for my first bottle and online classes. I found a diet that actually works and is the last diet I'll ever need. Meaning...I go on a strict diet for a few weeks, lose about a pound a day, and then take 3 weeks "setting" my new lower weight by eating more foods but no added sugar and no starches. Then I am set free. I had the whole summer off and went up 3 pounds above my lowest (at the time). Believe me, I ate whatever I wanted. I have 4 kids at home and I had ice cream almost everyday with them.

Then I found out that I have a local health food store that sells the same exact 2 oz. bottle for very little money, comparably.

You can try to get the drops locally. Call your local health food store and ask if they have hCG homeopathic drops. I'm in the Toledo, OH area, see the credits to find where to get a 2 ounce bottle for around $30.

As of March 2011, I have done 5 Rounds of the hCG diet. I average about 20 lbs each time. For a grand total loss of 80 lbs! I took last summer off, just in time for summer vacations. Sometimes my weight goes up a little, but the 'steak day' always works for me. My average is 6 days a week I get to eat anything I want and then one day a week, I "diet" or "fast" by having a "steak day".

My goal is to fit into a special pair of jeans I bought while on my honeymoon 14 years ago. After 5 Rounds of hCG diet, I now weigh 149, the lightest I've weighed in all my adult years. I'm 5'6½ and started out a size 20, and now wear a size 8. Loving the new clothes and those 100% hemp jeans from my honeymoon fit too! My "Post Weight Loss" photo was shown on The Dr. Oz Show, aired Monday January 3, 2011.

Update, I am maintained beautifully at the low to mid 150s for about three years, fitting into size 8 jeans. I had some health set back and let myself gain some weight. I am on the protocol as I type this to get back to a healthier for me size.

If you are looking for another book to read after this to delve into the topic of emotional eating and learning how to eat to the hunger scale, I highly recommend "Weight-Loss Apocalypse: Emotional Eating Rehab Through the hCG Protocol" by Robin Phipps Woodall. You can follow her youtube channel too.

I keep busy juggling being a mom of four children. My love of photography has been with me since I picked up a camera for 4H at age 12. Please check out my website when you get a chance. Prints are for sale directly from my site. www.scamperartistry.com
I like to use natural products and essential oils whenever I can. Like Sunrder and Melaleuca and Young Living products. I swear by the health benefits that drinking Shakeology daily has done for me. I have not been to the doctor in almost 3 years except for well check ups! I used to get shingles, and chest infections, sinus infections, strep throat, and stuff like that every year. I joined a Beachbody

Challenge, signing up as a coach to get the discount on Shakeology and now I help others achieve their fitness goals too. Visit beachbodycoach.com/lisabellison to find out more.

Find my facebook page titled "HCG Awesome - Success Secrets Revealed" to stay connected. Ask to join the private facebook group titled "Success Secrets Revealed - SCAMPER Artistry League". I spend a little more time on this facebook page, "Lisa B Ellison - Health and Fitness" lately. Find my blog at scamperartistry.blogspot.com

Best wishes on your weight-loss journey. Check with your doctor before starting any weight-loss or exercise program.

HCG Awesome

Success Secrets Revealed

To order a matching Route 66 theme weight-loss journal please visit
www.cafepress.com/hcgawesome

Compiled and self-published by
Lisa B. Ellison

SCAMPER Artistry Photography
www.scamperartistry.com

Credits

Anyana-Kai, 3344 Secor Rd., Toledo, OH 43606, ph. 419-720-2972 carries the 2 oz bottle. Their website is anyanakai.com.

hCG Miracle at www.hcgmiracle.com and on facebook. Online ordering and online classes and recipes with supportive message board.

Health Yourself, 10075 Fremont Pike, Perrysburg, OH 43551, Ph. 419-874-3355. Online ordering is here, healthyourselfalive.com/catalog. Health Yourself is very knowledgeable and friendly. They sell the 2 oz. bottle at the counter of their store. Their website is healthyourselfalive.com

Simply Total Health has the latest technology, great products. I wear the bracelets all the time and their "Simply ReSet" is what to take while on the protocol. They are on facebook and their website is www.simplytotalhealth.org

Shakeology – The Healthiest Meal Of The Day. Dense super nutrition daily. Website – shakeology.com/lisabellison

Maria Mind Body Health at www.marianutrition.com for inspiration from their healthful recipes found on their facebook page.

POUNDS AND INCHES Privately printed: obtainable only from A.T.W. Simeons, Salvator Mundi International Hospital, Rome, Italy
E.P. Dutton, New York (hardback) Dutton Paperbacks, New York

The Lighter Side of Low Carb, recipes found on their blog and on facebook.

Until the Thin Lady Sings: Gluten Free Low Carb Recipe Blog, blog and facebook page.

Please read the doctor's original manuscript is at the end of this book.

Questions and Answers

What is hCG?

hCG stands for "human chorionic gonadotrophin" - a hormone produced in very high quantities during pregnancy in women. During certain phases of pregnancy a woman may excrete as much as one million Internations Units per day in her urine.

What is homeopathic hCG?
Homeopathic hCG is produced by taking small amounts of the original hCG, and mixing it into a version that can be taken under the tongue (sublingually).

Does homeopathic hCG work as well as the hCG injections?
YES! We hear from many who have switched from hCG injections due to the cost and hassle with mixing the formula and poking themselves with needles. Homeopathic hCG works just as well, if not better.

Who can use this Weight Loss Cure?
Always check with your doctor before beginning any weight loss program. This treatment works for almost everyone, young, old, male, female, although we do not recommend hCG for anyone under age 18. We don't recommend using hCG if your BMI value is less than 20. We do not recommend using hCG if you are pregnant or nursing, or if you have had certain cancers that could be hormonally affected. If you have a history of gallstones there is an increased chance of having another episode. Check with your health care professional if you have had your gallbladder removed, or if you have autoimmunity, lupus, or inflammatory conditions. As we have always said, you should check with your health care professional before beginning any new weight loss program, especially if you have health conditions.

Will my birth control methods be affected by using hCG?
hCG will not interfere with any form of birth control.

Are there any side effects with using hCG
There are virtually no side effects associated with hCG. Very few experience slight headaches or dizziness for the first few days but this is extremely rare

and mild. HCG has been used for weight loss for 50+ years, so there is plenty of evidence to back up its safety. Dr. Simeons does state that teenage girls may, in some rare cases, experience delays or even interruptions to their cycle.

How many drops are recommended?
The nature of homeopathic is that they have a trace amount of the original substance, with a small but potent dosage. They work just as well as the prescription hCG, and some say, even better, because the extreme dilution of the substance actually enhances the curative properties. Homeopathies work on FREQUENCY of dose, not AMOUNT of dose. 6 drops, 6 times a day will keep the hCG in your system at a steady dose. If you wish to increase later we recommend you start by adding another dosage, 6 drops 7 times per day. Remember, it takes 72 hours for the new dosage of hCG to take effect.

How much hCG do I need to buy?
That depends on how much weight you have to lose. Average weight loss in women is approximately 1 1/2 pounds per day in the first week, and approximately 1/2 pound a day thereafter. Men usually lose more, and they lose it faster. The 30 Day Program with the 2 ounce bottle of hCG will last you approximately 30 days. If you need to lose more than that, go for the 40 Day Program.

Will the hCG interfere with medications my doctor has prescribed to me?
Homeopathies by nature are said to not interfere with prescriptions and we have not heard of any adverse reactions with any prescriptions, but please check with your prescribing physician.

Do I need to refrigerate the hCG?
Homeopathic hCG does not have to be refrigerated. It is mixed with alcohol, which acts as a preservative. The doctor we confer with says even an opened bottle will last for years. Just place it in a cool, dark place --- like your spice cupboard. Don't leave it in places where it can get hot, like your car in hot weather.

I don't have that much to lose. What is the shortest I can do the hCG program?
You MUST stay on the hCG for a MINIMUM of 23 days. If you reach your goal weight before you reach 23 days, you will simply increase your calories while still taking the hCG 23 days. Refer to VLCD for detailed instructions for ending your program correctly. By following this protocol you will reset the hypothalamus and keep the weight off FOREVER!

I have LOTS to lose. What is the longest I can do the hCG program?
Per Dr. Simeons' protocol, you may continue the hCG for a maximum of 40 days or 34 pounds - whichever comes first. Since hCG is homeopathic, if you are losing steadily at 40 days and have not reached 34 pounds you may choose to continue up to 60 days. Please refer VLCD for detailed instructions for ending your program correctly and for the rules on starting another round, if desired. By following Dr. Simeons' recommendations you will give your body a chance to rest between rounds.

How much weight can I expect to lose?
Weight loss varies and for women usually averages out to around 1 1/2 pound per day in the first week, and approximately 1/2 pounds per day thereafter. Men almost always lose more, and lose it faster.

Is it healthy to lose weight that fast?
With hCG - YES! You are losing fat - NOT muscle. And it is that stored fat that your body normally stubbornly holds on to!

Is it true that I won't feel like I am starving?
YES, it is true! While some do experience mild hunger during the first days, most do not. If you do experience hunger it will pass soon. Remember, your body is feeding off of thousands of calories per day - gloriously coming from your released fat!

Are there specific foods on the diet?
YES! You MUST eat ONLY from this list of foods. But no worries, all of the food on the list is REAL, NUTRITIOUS and easy to find in your supermarket. How wonderful to feel your body respond to these foods with ENERGY, VITALITY! Find the list under VCLD or in the Dr. Simeon's manuscript.

What sweeteners can I use on the program?
Sweetleaf Liquid Stevia is the preferred brand. (Some other brands have additives that actually contain sugar.) Aspartame, Nutrisweet, Acesulfame, Sucralose, and Splenda have been chemically and we don't recommend the use of any chemically derived sugar substitutes during this treatment.

Is it true that I don't need any additional supplements or vitamins while taking hCG?
Dr. Simeons states very emphatically that your blood will be saturated with vitamins and minerals released from your fat cells. He stresses that there is no need for additional supplements. This is why we only use hCG with NO added

supplements. If Dr. Simeons wanted us to take extra supplements, he would have said so in his "Pounds and Inches" manuscript. Don't be fooled by salespeople who want to push more products on you and do be careful, as some supplements can actually cause more harm than good. Of course, check with your health care professional regarding any supplements he has recommended to you before discontinuing their use.

Are there any restrictions as to when I should begin?
YES! Dr. Simeons is very clear. In menstruating women, the best time to start treatment is immediately after a period. Treatment may be started later, but have at least 10 days before the onset of the next period.

Where can I find melba toast, grissini breadsticks, stevia, and a food scale?
Melba toast can usually be found in your local grocery store in in the cracker aisle. Some grocers carry grissini in the Italian section, some in the cracker section, and some not at all. You may order it online at amazon.com. Liquid stevia can be found in many health food stores under the label "Sweetleaf" or order online at www.vitacost.com.. A scale can be found in most department stores - make sure you buy one small enough to weigh ounces - a letter scale works great.

Disclaimer: The products and the claims made about specific products on or through this site have not been evaluated by the United States Food and Drug Administration and are not approved to diagnose, treat, cure, or prevent disease. The information provided on this site is for informational purposes only, and it is not intended as a substitute for advice from your physician or other health care professional or any information contained on or in any label or packaging. You should not use the information on this site for diagnosis or treatment of any health problem or for prescription of any medication or other treatment. You should consult with a healthcare professional before starting any diet, exercise or supplementation program, before taking any medication, or if you suspect you might have a health problem.

Products
"Most women find it hard to believe that fats, oils, creams, and ointments applied to the skin are absorbed and interfere with weight reduction by HCG just as if they had been eaten. This almost incredible sensitivity to even such very minor increases in nutritional intake is a peculiar feature of the HCG method.* - Dr. ATW Simeons

It is not necessary to go out and replace all of your beauty/toiletry products! Many participants use many of their usual products. However, do replace your oil-based makeup and lotions, since those will be absorbed by the skin. Try to go foundation and lipstick free on the days you are home. Perhaps you can also get away with no deodorant when you are home. If you find your hands are getting extremely dry try baby oil (which is basically mineral oil) and gloves at night. And if you need to rub lotion or ointment into a young child you may want to don some gloves first. Pure natural coconut oil may also be used (with caution).

Do not use products containing oil while on the hCG protocol. While shopping for products, read labels. Some examples of products that can be used:

Face Soaps and Make-up Removers
Mineral or Baby Oil (great for removing leftover mascara around eyes)
Arbonne * All Botanical Based Skin Care
Neutrogena Deep Clean Cream Cleanser - Oil Free
Witch Hazel
Kiss My Face Wash, Toner, or Mask

Cosmetics
Any Oil-Free based Make-up/Foundation (read ingredients!)
Bare Essentials/Bare Minerals
Raw Minerals
Max Factor Pancake

Deodorants
Baking Soda
Crystalux or Thai Stick Crystal Deodorants
Crystal Deodorant Stick
Thai Deodorant Stick
Kiss My Face Liquid Rock
If you need more protection than the baking soda or crystal provide alone, use crystal first, then dust dry armpit with dry baking soda
Lotions/Moisturizers
Mineral or Baby Oil (if you have dry skin, apply at night to face, lips, hands)
Alba Oil Free Facial Moisturizer
Aloe Vera 100% Gel
Kiss My Face Oil Free Moisturizer or Eye Repair Creme
Neutrogena Oil Free Facial Moisture - for dry, oily, or combination skin

You may get VERY dry lips in the beginning of protocol and can find relief with a few applications of medicated Blistex. Use sparingly, but no need to walk around with cracked lips!

Detox Bath
1 - 2 cups of baking soda, and 1 - 2 cups of Epsom salt to the bathtub to soothe your skin while helping your body eliminate toxins. Heavenly!

Shampoos / Conditioners
Magick Botanicals Oil Free Shampoo and Conditioner (www.myvitanet.com)
Giovanni "50-50" or "Root 66" shampoo/conditioners - Walmart/Target
Life Extension (read label - some have oils)
Mastey Products (read label - some have oils)
Natures Gate Alovera

Soap
Dial
Ivory
Jason's
Zest
Baking Soda
Kiss My Face Organic Foaming Liquid Soap

Sunscreens
Aveeno Oil Free Sunscreen
Clarins Oil Free Sun Care Spray SPF 15
Copportone Oil Free Sun Block for Faces SPF 30
Copportone Oil Free Sun Block Lotion
Oil Free Sport Xtreme Sun Block
Peter Thomas Roth Ultra Lite Oil Free sun products
Zia Oil Free Sunscreen SPF 15

Toothpastes
Baking Soda
Arm & Hammer Baking Soda & Peroxide
Spry Toothpaste
Tom's of Maine Toothpaste

Homeopathic Drops

For best results follow the instructions on your own bottle.
The following is an example of instructions.

hCG Homeopathic Drops
Do not eat or drink for 15 minutes before or after taking the hCG.
Homeopathic should be taken on a clean palate. Strong flavors, such as coffee
or toothpaste, can disrupt the working of a remedy. Give your bottle a gentle
swirl before opening. Open, release the liquid in the dropper back into the
bottle, re-load, and, while watching yourself in the mirror, slowly release 6
drops under your tongue.

Now count, slowly, to 15 seconds minimum ... but let's shoot for 30 seconds,
or more, if you prefer. Then swallow. Take note of the time. Remember, do
not drink or eat anything for a minimum of 15 minutes.

Take 6 drops, 6 times a day, spaced evenly throughout your day. For instance,
8 am, 11 a.m., 2 p.m., 5 p.m., 8 p.m., 11 p.m.

Store your drops in a dark, cool location. They do not need to be refrigerated.
Don't leave them somewhere they can heat up --- like your car on a hot day.
Do keep them in a little bubble bag, or in another protective container, even
when you take them - just in case you drop your bottle!

RECAP:
6 drops 6 times daily
Space evenly throughout day
Store in dark, cool location
Don't need to be refrigerated
Don't leave in hot car
Do use a little bubble-wrap bag just in case you drop it

LOADING – The first two days of taking the drops

Now, for the fun stuff. For two days, starting the first day you take your drops, you are to eat the fattiest foods you can. Lots of heavy cream in your coffee. Deep fried, rich, creamy, fattening foods. Heavy cream in your coffee, or in a shake. Cheesecake. Fast food is great. French fries. Onion rings. Ice cream. Chocolate. Whip cream. Chips with dips. Mayo. Butter. Cream cheese. Deep fried mozzarella sticks. Have fun--no kidding!

Concentrate on the FAT. It's not about loading as much food as you can ~ it's about loading as much FAT as you can. So avoid filling up on starches ~ load up on FAT.

You are loading fat to ensure that your NORMAL fat is sufficient, and to help you feel more comfortable through the first week of the Very Low Calorie Diet.

Try this healthy coconut oil "fat bombs" recipe:
1 cup coconut oil (melted)
1 cup almond butter
1 cup chocolate Shakeology
1/3 to 1/2 cup local honey

Mix it all together and pour into small ice cube trays or the plastic top of egg cartons. Freeze, pop into mouth. Store in airtight container in freezer.

PREPARE

Record your Before measurements. Have a notebook ready to record your daily weight. You will need to weigh yourself completely naked right after going to the bathroom, first thing in the morning.

Consider having some supplies ready:
Sweetleaf liquid Stevia ~ health food stores or www.vitacost.com

Capella flavor drops ~ flavor your water with orange mango, peach, cherry, et. www.capellaflavordrops.com

Natural Bristle Brush ~ found at most department stores ~ great for exfoliating dry skin

Letter scale ~ in 1 oz increments ~ found at many department stores (Walmart $20)

Weight scale ~ in 1 oz increments

Oil-free personal care products ~ see list in "Safe Products"

Mineral or Baby oil

Coffee, Tea, Green Tea

Melba Toast Classic (no variations, as they contain oil!) or Grissino Bread Sticks ~ melba is in cracker aisle, grissino may be in cracker or pasta section, or ordered online

Veal, Beef, Chicken Breast, Fresh White Fish, Lobster, Crab, Shrimp

Spinach, Chard, Chicory, Beet-greens, Green Salad, Tomatoes, Celery, Fennel, Onions, Red Radishes, Cucumbers, Asparagus, Cabbage

Apple, Orange, Strawberries, or Grapefruit

Lemons ~ get a bag!

Sugar-Free Seasonings

Take the drops for a minimum of 23 days and starting on day 3 and continuing starts the VLCD.

THE VERY LOW CALORIE DIET aka VLCD

The following is straight out of Dr. Simeons' Pounds & Inches Manuscript

* *

Breakfast:
Tea or coffee in any quantity without sugar. Only one tablespoonful of milk allowed in 24 hours.

Lunch:
1) 100 grams (3 1/2 oz) of veal, beef, chicken breast, fresh white fish, lobster, crab or shrimp. All visible fat must be carefully removed before cooking, and the meat must be weighed raw. It must be boiled or grilled without additional fat. Salmon, eel, tuna, herring, dried or pickled fish are not allowed. The chicken breast must be removed raw from the bird.

2) One type of vegetable only to be chosen from the following: spinach, chard, chicory, beet-greens, green salad, tomatoes, celery, fennel, onions, red radishes, cucumbers, asparagus, cabbage.

3) One breadstick (grissino), or one melba toast

4) One apple, or an orange, or a handful of strawberries, or one-half grapefruit

Dinner:
The same four choices as lunch.

"The juice of one lemon daily is allowed for all purposes. Salt, pepper, vinegar, mustard powder, garlic, sweet basil, parsley, thyme, marjoram, etc., may be used for seasoning, but no oil, butter or dressing.

Tea, coffee, plain water, or mineral water are the only drinks allowed, but they may be taken in any quantity and at all times.

In fact, the patient should drink about 2 liters of these fluids per day. Many patients are afraid to drink so much because they fear that this may make them retain more water. This is a wrong notion as the body is more inclined to store water when the intake falls below its normal requirements.

The fruit or the breadstick may be eaten between meals instead of with lunch or dinner, but not more than four items listed for lunch and dinner may be eaten at one meal.

The 100 grams of meat must he scrupulously weighed raw after all visible fat has been removed.

To do this accurately the patient must have a letter-scale, as kitchen scales are not sufficiently accurate and the butcher should certainly not be relied upon.

Every item in the list is gone over carefully, continually stressing the point that no variations other than those listed may be introduced.

Those not uncommon patients who feel that even so little food is too much for them, can omit anything they wish.

All things not listed are forbidden, and the patient is assured that nothing permissible has been left out.

No medicines or cosmetics other than lipstick, eyebrow pencil and powder may be used without special permission. "

~ Dr. Simeons, Pounds & Inches Manuscript

HOW MUCH IS 100 GRAMS?
100 grams = 3 1/2 ounces. You will need that scale we mentioned in Class 1 to weigh your meat. A letter scale is the most accurate. Weigh meat RAW - before cooking.

SHOULD I COUNT MY CALORIES?
After researching this question carefully, we suggest that you do, at least in the first week of your VLCD. Here's what Dr. Simeons says about calories in his Pounds and Inches Manuscript:

"The diet, used in conjunction with hCG must not exceed 500 Calories per day, and the way these Calories are made up is of utmost importance. For instance, if a patient drops the apple and eats an extra breadstick instead, he will not be getting more Calories but he will not lose weight." ~ Dr. Simeons

Further in his manuscript, he states,

. . . "the total daily intake must not exceed 500 Calories if the best possible results are to be obtained, (and) that the daily ration should contain 200 grams of fat-free protein and a very small amount of starch."

3 1/2 ounces of beef has more calories than 3 1/2 ounces of chicken, fish, or seafood. If you have steak for one meal you are going to need to watch your calories for the rest of your foods that day, and perhaps consider fish/seafood for your other meal.

CHEATING

Please remember that this is not a diet that you can cheat on. This is a CURE. But you must follow Dr. Simeons' instructions precisely. Make a VOW to yourself that you will give 100% to this program. Make a vow that you will not take one taste or one sip of anything that is not on the program. You may think you got away with it when you weigh-in after a cheat, but you may have trouble stabilizing your weight during and after Maintenance. Give this GIFT of a CURE to yourself. Give 100% and you will get back 100%!

This is what Dr. Simeons says in his Pounds & Inches manuscript,

"It is impressed upon him that he will have to follow the prescribed diet to the letter ... ... If these conditions are not acceptable the case is refused, as any compromise or half-measure is bound to prove utterly disappointing to patient and physician alike and is a waste of time and energy.

WATER, WATER, WATER

Drinking water is very important to your SUCCESS in both taking weight off during VLCD, and maintaining your weight loss later. In fact, we have found that the weight loss is GREATER during the VLCD when the body is fully hydrated. Shoot for one-half your body's weight in ounces of water, up to 100 ounces or so. Did you know that if you drink with a straw you take in about 25% more water? Add some sliced lemon. Or make a little lemonade, with water, lemon juice, lemon, and stevia. Drink up, everybody!

HEADACHES

Some starting out find themselves with a headache for a few days, some do not. Your body may be reacting to a sugar withdrawal. Or, perhaps you quit drinking your favorite coffee drink, and you are experiencing a caffeine withdrawal. It is fine to take aspirin. And usually a cup of coffee with that aspirin will help. If you don't care for black coffee consider replacing it with green tea, or herbal teas. Or check out the Recipes link for some on-protocol yummy blended coffee drinks. If you do cut out caffeine altogether than take our advice, and wean yourself off slowly to avoid the headache. .

POTTY TALK

It is normal for your bowel movements to slow way down, as you take in such low calories in food. During the start of VLCD have a little Smooth Move Tea, if you haven't "unloaded" the "loading" days food. After that, there is no need to be concerned but you may certainly have a cup or two of Smooth Move Tea again, to get things moving. Smooth Move Tea can be found at many grocers, or in your health food store. Please do not over-use the Smooth Move Tea, as your body can become reliant on it. Dr. Simeons actually prefers a laxative in the form of a suppository, so if the Smooth Move Tea isn't cutting it, we recommend you go that route.

DETOX BATH

Take a relaxing bath ~ soften your skin ~ and detox at the same time! Just add 1-2 cups Epsom salt and 1-2 cups baking soda to your bathtub. Light a candle, and enjoy!

WEIGHING

Weigh yourself naked every morning after using the bathroom. Weigh in at the same time each morning, when possible. Do not eat or drink anything before you weigh in. Your weight loss is going to be the most dramatic in the first week to ten days. After that, the weight loss will likely slow down to an average of one half to one pound a day. You will also experience a stall. This is norma.

STALLS

Your weight, in almost every case, will stall for a few days at some point or two during your round. Please remember that this is NORMAL. We always recommend that you do a REVIEW of EVERYTHING any time that your weight slows down, just in case.

Review:
Did you eat/drink/do anything different?
Did your hands come in contact with oils/fats/creams?
Did you drink enough water?
Did you take any medicines that contain sugar?
Is that time of the month approaching, or here?

Were you hCG doses evenly spaced?
Do you have a cold? (Yes, Dr. S. says that may cause a weight gain!)
Did you over-exert yourself the day before, to the point of exhaustion?
Are you getting enough sleep?

After reviewing, tweak any changes that may need to be made, and carry on.
Your weight loss WILL resume and meanwhile, you are still releasing FAT,
every single day. If you took your measurements at the beginning this is a
good time to re-measure, and see just how far you've come.

A PLATEAU can last for 4-6 days, and frequently occurs during the second
half of a round, particularly in patients that have been doing well and whose
overall weight loss average of nearly a pound per day has been maintained.
Those who are losing more than the average ALL have a plateau sooner or
later. Again, do a REVIEW of EVERYTHING, just in case. A plateau always
corrects itself so try to RELAX and let the hCG work its magic. Dr. Simeons
does offer you an *Apple Day* if you are just getting too anxious about the
plateau.

APPLE DAY: Begins at lunch and continues until just before lunch of the
following day. You may eat up to six large apples. Drink just enough water to
quench an "uncomfortable" thirst. No other foods or liquids are allowed.

REACHING A FORMER LEVEL is another possible cause for stalls of ten
days to two weeks. This is rare and only occurs in very advanced cases and
hardly ever during the first round. This can occur when you reach a weight
that you were at for several years. Do your REVIEW of EVERYTHING. Try
to RELAX, knowing that your weight loss WILL resume.

TIME of MONTH (TOM) is another culprit for stalls that we see in most
women and occurs a few days before and during the menstrual cycle and in
some women, at the time of ovulation. Again, try to RELAX * this is
NORMAL and your weight loss will resume soon

Remember, even if the scale is not budging, you can rest assured that the
inches are!

FAT is being extracted from your cells daily
When these cells EMPTY, they take a while to break down in the body

They may fill with water - temporarily - which can account for bit of a stall, or even gain, on the scale
When they do empty you will see the scale drop again

EXERCISE
Only mild exercise is allowed during the VLCD stage of this program. You just don't have enough calories or protein to do more than that. Walking and swimming are the two exercises that Dr. Simeons recommends. In fact, he also says that you may GAIN WEIGHT "after an exceptional physical exertion of long duration that leads to the point of exhaustion." from overexerting yourself. And yes, that includes hard physical labor. So take a walk and enjoy the break. We encourage you to exercise more after the VLCD.

CONSTIPATION
Do not expect to have a bowel movement every day. On the VLCD it is more common to have one every three or four days. Dr. Simeons does not allow laxatives except in the form of a suppository, and only in patients who have gone more than four days without a bowel movement and are getting anxious about it.

hCG DOSAGE
6 drops, 6 times a day is the recommended dosage from the FDA approved laboratory that makes our hCG. It is also the recommended dosage of our consulting doctor that runs an hCG Weight Loss Center.

If anyone is telling you that you need to double the amount of hCG drops to "equal the IUs of injectable hCG" they simply do not know understand the nature of homeopathic. You cannot "match" the dosage of injectable hCG with homeopathic. Homeopathic don't work that way!

The nature of homeopathic is that they have a trace amount of the original substance, with a small but potent dosage. The dosage varies according to each homeopathic product. The laboratory determines the dosage based on the potency they created, and the function it must perform in the human body.

Homeopathic work on FREQUENCY of dosing. Frequency is more important than the amount. In fact, you could take a entire bottle of homeopathic hCG 6 times a day, and it would have the same weight loss effect as your 6 drop dosage!

SUPPLEMENTS
We want to advise you to use CAUTION when considering supplements.
Many sites are going to try to "upsell" you their products. Dr. Simeons was
very clear that we receive all the nutrients that we need from the released fat,
and his diet is full of nutritious, real foods, high in vitamins and nutrients. We
use pure hCG with no additives or supplements. Taking certain supplements
may indeed be necessary, but they can also be harmful for some people who
may have underlying health conditions. Every body is different, so ask your
health care professional what is right for YOU.

For instance, potassium. Symptoms of low levels of potassium are similar to
symptoms of high levels of potassium - both include fatigue, muscle weakness,
and heart palpitations. And too much potassium can be just as dangerous as
too little. We recommend that you check with your health care professional
before taking potassium supplements. Dr. Simeons has many foods on the
VLCD that are naturally RICH in potassium: chard, spinach, fennel, kale,
tomato, cucumber, strawberries, halibut, cabbage, cod, and oranges. Be sure to
eat them on a regular basis. You may also use dried seasonings, such as: basil,
parsley, turmeric, and ginger, to increase your potassium levels naturally.

Again, use CAUTION - and ask your health care professional what is right for
YOU - when considering adding supplements to your diet.

WHEN YOU DECIDE IT IS TIME TO MOVE ON TO MAINTENANCE,
PLEASE REMEMBER...
*Dr. Simeons protocol is to stay on the hCG a minimum of 23 days
*Dr. Simeons protocol is to discontinue use of the hCG at a maximum of 40
days OR 34 pounds, whichever comes first.
*Since this hCG is homeopathic you *may* choose to go longer than 40 days
if you have not yet reached 34 lbs.
*The maximum recommendation for homeopathic hCG is 60 days.

WHEN YOU ARE READY TO STOP TAKING THE HCG ...
First, consider your cycle. Dr. Simeons states that the end of a course of hCG
should never be made to coincide with menstruation. If it happens to work out
that way, it's better to give the last dose three days before the expected date of
your period, so that a normal diet can be resumed when it is over. Or, as an
alternative, at least three doses should be given after the period, followed by
the three days of no hCG with the VLCD. Remember, Dr. Simeons was

referring to injectable hCG doses, which is given once daily. So three doses actually means three days after the period.

(*If you have already reached your goal weight before the end of your drops and have already been on a higher calorie diet, you need not concern yourself with the above.)

Second, you MUST still continue the vlcd for 72 hours after the last dose. That's how long it takes the hCG to leave your system. Stop the hCG. Chart your weight the morning of your last dose - this is your "Last Drop Weight", or LDW. Continue the vlcd diet for 72 hours after your last dosage. You will be comfortable, as the hCG is still in your system. You may notice that you begin to get hungry during those last few hours, as you are no longer releasing fat into your system without the hCG. We were comfortable throughout.

After 72 hours free from hCG . . . you will be off to Maintenance

MAINTENANCE

THE HYPOTHALAMUS
The hypothalamus is, in Dr. Simeons' words, "the part from which the central nervous system controls all the automatic animal functions of the body, such as breathing, the heart beat, digestion, sleep, sex, the urinary system, the autonomous or vegetative nervous system and via the pituitary the whole interplay of the endocrine glands."

As you can see, this is a very delicate and sensitive part of our brain. That's why it is SO important that we follow Dr. Simeons instructions, exactly.

MAINTENANCE PROTOCOL
"When the three days of dieting after the last injection are over, the patients are told that they may now eat anything they please, except sugar and starch provided they faithfully observe one simple rule." ~ Dr. S

Dr. S's Golden Rule:
"This rule is that they must have their own portable bathroom-scale always at hand, particularly while traveling. They must without fail weight themselves every morning as they get out of bed, having first emptied their bladder." If you gain more over 2 pounds, even by a few ounces, you must immediately correct it with a Steak Day - that day!

STEAK DAY
"Skip breakfast and lunch but take plenty to drink. In the evening eat a huge steak with only an apple or a tomato." ~ Dr. S

Maintenance is 21 days.

Why 3 weeks of Maintenance?
"It takes about 3 weeks before the weight reached at the end of the treatment becomes stable, i.e. does not show violent fluctuations after an occasional excess." ~ Dr. S

What do I avoid?
"During this period patients must realize that the so-called carbohydrates, that are sugar, rice, bread, potatoes, pastries etc, are by far the most dangerous." ~ Dr. S

Dr. Simeons kept it pretty simple, didn't he? We suggest you follow his lead, and do the same.

But how do I determine starches and sugars in foods?

NO SUGAR - read INGREDIENTS on EVERYTHING because sugar is added to so many items. Remember, you are looking for sugar in the list of INGREDIENTS. If there is no added sugar, but the NUTRITION LABEL shows sugar, then it's a natural sugar, which is fine.

Tomatoes have natural sugar, for instance ... so if a tomato sauce does not list sugar in the INGREDIENTS, but does list sugar in the NUTRITION LABEL, you are just fine. If it contains less than 2% of sugar in the ingredients, you are to use "caution" with that food, but may be fine with a small serving.

NO STARCH - again, reading ingredients on EVERYTHING because certain starches are added to many foods; i.e., potato starch.

For starchy foods a great resource is www.nutritiondata.com. At the top right of the screen you will see a box to type in the food, then enter the category for that food. When the nutrition data appears, adjust the serving size. Then scroll down and you'll find a box that shows the amount of carbohydrates and starch.

Some key words to watch for in your ingredients: flour, wheat, rye, barley, oats, oatmeal, spelt, millet, hydrolyzed wheat protein, sprouted wheat, barley malt, high-gluten flour, vital gluten, wheat gluten, bulgur, durum, farina, mochi, matzo, matza, kamut, graham, semolina, triticum.

Anything with the words: sugar, syrup, sweetener, juice, and all words ending in *ose*; honey, molasses, brown rice syrup, treacle, turbinado, maltodextrin, destrin.

It is the combination of avoiding sugars/starches and not gaining more than 2 pounds during the 21 days that resets the hypothalamus.

It is also important to note that - if the VLCD and Maintenance are followed correctly - the hypothalamus will reset to the weight you saw on the scale the morning of the last day you took HCG. We refer to this as the LDW (last drop weight).

So, if you weigh 150 on the day of your last dose of hCG, but then go and lose another 5 pounds during the 21-days (which is not recommended), the hypothalamus will reset at 150 pounds not 145.

So, what can I eat?
Yes, let's discuss all the delicious foods that you may now add in to your menu.

NOTE: Some foods are "cautionary", meaning, you should use caution with both quantity and frequency, and you should not combine too many 'cautionary" foods in one day.

PROTEINS
Meat: All meats! All seafood! All fish! (except caviar) Even bacon (a few slices, not a pound)! Processed meats like hot dogs, pepperoni, beef jerky are cautionary and are not advised in the first week of Maintenance, but all other meats are now open to you. Yippee!!
Eggs: Yes!
Milk: Yes, but use caution with the amount of milk. And avoid any milks with added sugar (as in some soy/rice milks).
Cheese: Yes, but use caution with the amount of cheese, and read labels. Shredded cheeses usually contain starches so that they won't stick in the package. Shred your own. - and use caution in the amount used.

Increase your animal/egg protein from vlcd portions to normal portions now, and eat a protein at each of 3 meals per day. A boiled egg or two for breakfast. A regular sized boneless, skinless chicken breast. A normal size steak. A hamburger patty. A pork chop. Tuna fish packed in water with a little mayo on your salad, or scooped up in celery. Etc.

Add more protein variety. After the VLCD your body is borderline protein deficient. It was not in any distress during VLCD because your blood stream was saturated with nutrients released from the fat cells. However, after the three days, when you are slowly eliminating the hCG from your system, your body no longer has the nutrients supplied by the hCG released fat and thus requires much more protein.

IMPORTANT: If you do not eat enough PROTEIN your body will begin to retain water. You will rapidly put on weight. And THAT makes some want to reduce their food further, which only contributes to more water retention.
FRUITS and VEGETABLES

Veggies: You may now add more variety to your vegetables. And yes, you can combine them. Hooray! Avoid starchy vegetables, like potatoes, corn, cooked beets, cow peas, yam,. Avoid pearl onions and tomato puree. Use caution with artichoke (hearts are fine), bamboo shoots, burdock root, shitake mushrooms, cooked okra, canned hearts of palm, green peas, canned pumpkin, and squash.

Fruits: Oh those glorious, glorious fruits are open to you once again! Do limit fruits to a maximum of two per day in the first week. Use caution with very sweet fruits like bananas, grapes, melons, prunes, pomegranates, raisins. Avoid dried cranberries, maraschino cherries, banana chips, canned cranberry sauce,

What about fats ... and alcohol?
"If no carbohydrates whatsoever are eaten, fats can be indulged in somewhat more liberally and even small quantities of alcohol, such as a glass of wine with meals, does no harm, but as soon as fat and starch are combined things are very liable to get out of hand. This has to be observed very carefully during the first 3 weeks after the treatment is ended otherwise disappointments are almost sure to occur." ~Dr. S

HEALTHY FATS
Add healthy fats to your diet . . . but go S-L-O-W-L-Y! Fats can be indulged in, "somewhat more liberally," remember? THIS IS NOT LOADING! Enjoy a few slices of avocado. Have a little real cream in your coffee, if you wish. Spread a tablespoon of all-natural, no-sugar peanut butter on your apple slices. Use a tablespoon or two of real sugar-free mayonnaise or salad dressing on your salad. READ LABELS. If it contains sugar, is NOT for Maintenance. Nuts are cautionary, a little handful will do..

ALCOHOL
We don't recommend alcohol during your first week of Maintenance. After that hard alcohol (vodka, whiskey, rum, tequila, gin, etc.) is cautionary, as are wines (no sweet wines though). Of course, be careful that you don't drink them with liquids that contain sugar. Sorry, beer is not being served at this time. Cheers!

What about snacks, and desserts?
We don't recommend eating processed foods during your first week of
Maintenance. After that, please, use caution. Try ONE serving of ONE new
item, and see how it affects your weight. Some cautionary snacks and desserts
are: sugar-free jello, sugar-free popsicles, sugar-free dreamsicles, sugar-free
creamsicles, sugar-free fudgecicles, etc. Fat-free/sugar-free vanilla frozen
yogurt. f you are craving cereal, start with a small serving of puffed millet but
use caution with the milk - if you mix a little milk with water it will go further.

What about diet beverages?
We suggest you hold off during your first week of Maintenance. Also think
about the chemicals in diet beverages, and whether or not you really want to
pour them back in to your newly cleansed body. We don't really know how/if
those chemicals will affect you during this delicate time of rebalancing.
Ultimately, it's your decision.

How about my grissini and Melba toast?
Nope. Grissini and Melba toast are starches, and we are avoiding starches
during Maintenance.

Okay, but I'm afraid if I eat "normal" portions of even just "real" food I will
gain the weight back!
In addition to Dr. S's "2 Pound Rule" we suggest that, when you see the scale
creep up, you do a "5 Step Review". (Note: this is when the scale creeps up,
NOT when you are over your 2.2 lb limit!)

5 Step Review:

1. Review what you may have done differently the day before
2. Analyze what you ate, drank, and any other factors that may be in play
3. Re-adjust anything that you find that needs tweaking
4. Ignore gains due to TOM or medications that are not "true weight" gains
(i.e., you KNOW without a doubt that this cannot POSSIBLY be from what
you ate the day before, and TOM has arrived, or you have taken a medication
that contained sugar.)
5. Carry on with Maintenance, but GO LEAN without any cautionary foods,
to bring your weight back down again. Plenty of lean protein and plain
veggies, with perhaps one fruit, will bring your weight back down again.

The "2 Pound Rule" and the additional "5 Step Review" will help you keep your weight in check during Maintenance.

But let's read what else Dr. Simeons says about eating normally in Maintenance...

"Some patients cannot believe that they can eat fairly normally without regaining weight. They disregard the advice to eat anything they please except sugar and starch and want to play safe. They try more or less to continue the 500-calorie diet on which they felt so well during treatment and make only minor variations, such as replacing the meat with an egg, cheese, or a glass of milk. To their horror they find that in spite of this bravura, their weight goes up." ~ Dr. S

Lori was so used to dieting all of her life that she - fresh from vlcd - was afraid that if she ate more, she would gain back the weight she lost during the vlcd. We've all been so disappointed by diet after diet, knowing that once we finished a diet we usually ballooned right up when we so much as looked at normal portions again. Well, Lori, afraid to eat normally, didn't increase her protein. She kept to small portions. And her body reacted by bloating up - fast. Her ankles were swollen. She couldn't think straight. So, watching that scale go up, she ate even less. She almost ended up in the hospital. Read her story...

"For people like me with serious weight problems, going from 500 calories to a NORMAL diet is very scary, and many people, like me, still think that eating less is better. Not so in the case of this protocol. I have never eaten 3 meals a day, and now I need to, and I almost landed myself in the hospital last night before I realized it. That transition is CRITICAL and scary, and people have to NOT be afraid to get all that food in. It IS a lot of food, but it's good nutritional, REAL food and it's not going to hurt the body like our old eating habits did. "

Should you find yourself with swollen ankles and retaining water, Dr. Simeons stresses that YOU NEED PROTEIN. You are to immediately do a "Steak and Cheese Day."

STEAK AND CHEESE DAY
Two eggs at breakfast, a huge steak at lunch and again at dinner, followed by a large helping of cheese. You will likely be up during the night as your body happily eliminate excess water. Lori did just that. She eliminated out

approximately 7 pounds of excess water. She learned a huge lesson - good nutritional REAL food is not going to hurt the body.

After 3 weeks of Maintenance, you can move into Maintenance 2 phase.

MAINTENANCE phase 2

"After 3 weeks, very gradually add starch in small quantities, always controlled by morning weighing."

This phase lasts 3 weeks. Sample foods that you are re-introducing into your diet. One slice of bread…wait until the next morning weigh in to see how it affects your body. If you decide you'd rather stick with the Maintenance 1 phase for longer, that's fine…but when you decide to add starches and sugars, you must do it slowly…doing 3 weeks Maintenance 2 phase.

Remember, any day the scale is 2 pounds plus a few ounces or more over your LDW (last drops weight), THAT DAY is The Steak Day. Drink plenty of fluids, eat nothing until evening, at which time you have a large steak and either a tomato or an apple.

LIFE

After the M1 and M2, you may start Round 2. After each Round, you will add 2 more weeks of "Life" before starting another Round.
The last round the doctor mentions is that we need 6 months of "life" (after finishing maintenance 1 and 2) between round 5 and 6.

THIS IS YOUR RULE FOR THE REST OF YOUR LIFE.

THIS IS HOW YOU WILL KEEP THE WEIGHT OFF --- FOREVER!

VLCD Recipes

BEVERAGES

Strawberry or Orange Julius
1 cup crushed ice
1 cup partially defrosted Strawberries or 1 medium Orange
5 drops Orange Stevia
5 drops Vanilla Cream Stevia
Blend until smooth

Iced Java
3 - 5 ice cubes (not too many! it's not good if it's too thick)
vanilla creme stevia drops, to taste
1 Tbsp milk
if desired, add sprinkle of spice (cinnamon, pumpkin, etc)
1 cup of strong coffee
Mix in blender until frothy. Pour into glass and serve.

Ice-Cubed Java
Strong coffee, cooled, poured into ice cube trays, and frozen
chocolate or vanilla creme stevia drops, to taste
1 Tbsp milk
if desired, add sprinkle of spice (cinnamon, pumpkin, etc)
In blender mix 4-5 cubes of coffee, 1 Tbsp milk, and stevia. Add more water if needed for desired consistency.

Frozen Cappuccino
1 cup crushed ice
5 drops of peppermint stevia
5 drops of chocolate stevia
5 drops of Valencia orange
1 cup of coffee
Mix in blender until smooth. Pour into glass and serve.

Strawberry Smoothie
1 cup crushed ice
handful fresh strawberries
(or 1 cup water and handful of frozen strawberries)
vanilla creme stevia, to taste
1/2 lemon, juiced
Mix in blender and enjoy.

Lemon Drop Slushy
1/2 tsp. fresh squeezed lemon juice
1/2 cup water
1/2 cup ice
stevia, to taste
Mix in blender until slushy

DRESSINGS, BROTHS, SAUCES

Vinaigrette
1/3 cup apple cider vinegar
2 T. water
2 T. dried thyme
1/4 t. salt
1/4 t. pepper
1 T. dried basil
1/4 t. garlic powder
Add all ingredients in a blender and mix well.

Citrus Dressing
1/4 cup apple cider vinegar
1 cup water
1 T lemon
stevia to taste
1/4 t garlic powder

Dill Dressing
1/3 cup apple cider vinegar
2 T. water
2 T. dried basil
2 T. dried dill
1 t. garlic powder
1 t. dry mustard
1 t. onion powder
Mix all ingredients in a blender and mix well.

Vinaigrette Dressing
1/4 c. apple cider vinegar
1/2 c. water
2 shakes celery salt
2 shakes onion salt
Ground pepper to taste
stevia, to taste

Strawberry Vinaigrette Dressing
Strawberries
1 Tbsp apple cider vinegar
1 Tbsp lemon juice
stevia, to taste
dash of salt and dash of cayenne (optional)
fresh ground pepper, to taste
Combine all ingredients in food processor. Puree until smooth. Pour over fresh arugula or green salad. Garnish with sliced strawberries and freshly cracked pepper. Variation: use as marinate or sauce for chicken.

Chicken Broth
1 chicken breast
8 cups water
4 cups water
5 t. poultry season (no sugar)
5 t. onion powder
4 garlic cloves
4 t. black pepper
3 t. sea salt
3 T. celery salt
1 cheese cloth

1 string

Mix all herbs and place in the cheese cloth wrap string around cloth to secure all herbs and place it in the stock pot with 8 cups of water and the chicken breast and boil for 35 minutes or until chicken breast is cooked. Place a strainer on top of a bowl with a coffee filter to Strain broth to extract any fat from chicken breast and use the chicken for other recipes. Keep the cheese cloth to see if you need to continue to add more flavors to the stock for the additional 4cups of water and bring to a boil for additional 30 minutes. Set aside and chill. Use the broth for recipes for flavor and for a cup of broth before lunch and dinner.

APPETIZERS, SIDES, SALADS AND SOUPS

Citrus Shrimp & Greens
3.5 oz shrimp
2 Tbsp lemon juice
3 Tbsp apple cider vinegar
1 tsp garlic powder
1 tsp pepper
1/2 tsp onion salt

Mix ingredients together and then add shrimp. Let marinate for 1/2 hour. Grill shrimp or cook in hot non-stick frying pan. Serve over your favorite salad greens.

Crunchy Apple Chicken Salad
3.5 oz chicken, cooked and diced
1 apple, diced
3 stalks celery, diced
3 T lemon juice
1/8 t cinnamon
dash of nutmeg
dash of cardamom
dash of salt
stevia to taste
wedge of lemon

Mix ingredients together, sprinkle with stevia and cinnamon. Chill for 20 minutes. Serve with a wedge of lemon and enjoy. Maintenance modification: Add chopped walnuts or raw almonds. Mix in 1 T mayonnaise for a creamier texture.

Beet Greens or Asparagus

1 cup chicken broth (read label!)
1 cup chopped beet greens or asparagus
Dash of onion salt
Heat chicken broth & water on medium to just prior to boiling, Reduce heat, add greens and sauté a few minutes until tender. Sprinkle with onion salt.

Chicken Soup

3 1/2 oz raw chicken breast
1 bay leaf
fresh ground pepper, to taste
1 tsp parsley
dash sea salt
"large handful" favorite protocol vegetable (cabbage, spinach, diced tomatoes, or celery)
Place chicken breast in medium saucepan. Fill pan halfway with water. Add seasonings. Bring to boil. Reduce heat to simmer, cooking until chicken is done. Add vegetable. Shred chicken and return to pan. Continue simmering 30 minutes, covered. If using tomatoes throw them in at the start for a richer broth ... use 1/2 can sugar-free canned tomatoes, if desired. GREAT in a thermos for an easy and hot lunch at work!

Chicken Little's Meatballs and Spinach Soup

1 lb ground lean chicken breast (made into 1 inch balls)
8 cups water
1/2 tsp. garlic powder
1/2 tsp. onion salt
1/2 tsp. celery salt
1/2 tsp poultry seasoning
1/4 tsp fresh cracked pepper
1 * tsp sea salt
1 tsp turmeric
1 Tbsp chives
1 Tbsp parsley (fresh or dried)
2 tsp Mrs. Dash
1 whole bag fresh spinach
Mix all of the seasonings together in the pot, then add spinach. After spinach has cooked down gently add chicken, so that they do not break apart. Do not stir until the chicken has cooked a little bit to hold its shape. Adjust any of the seasonings per your taste. 1 pound ground chicken breast makes around 20-21

balls, and for 100 grams you may have 5. This recipes makes 4 servings, so you can refrigerate the leftovers and have another day's meal. Enjoy! It is very Yummy!

Chicken & Tomato Soup
3 1/2 ounce chicken breast
1/2 can S&W diced tomatoes with garlic, oregano & basil seasoning (not added chopped veggies)
pepper
parsley flakes

Place 2 cups water, chicken, tomatoes, and seasonings in a medium saucepan. Cook until chicken is tender and pulls apart easily. Remove chicken, shred, and add back to pan. Simmer a few minutes more. Enjoy!

French Onion Soup
1 Vidalia onion
2 c. beef broth (read label!)
3.5 ounces lean steak
1t. garlic powder
1t. onion salt
1t. pepper
2 Melba toast
Slice onion with an apple slicer to make wedges, and to open up the onion. Season the onion and place it on top of a foil sheet. Add 1?4 c beef broth, and wrap it up tightly, and place in a baking dish and bake at 350 degrees for 1 hour. You want to make sure the onion is not too soft you want it a little firm. Serve in a bowl with 2 cups of beef broth, sliced cooked steak, and 2 Melba toast.

Shrimp Soup
2 cups water
3 1/2 oz frozen shrimp
"handful" of shredded cabbage
Cajun seasoning (McCormick no-sugar)
garlic salt
Add shrimp and cabbage to water in a medium sauce pan. Add Cajun to taste. Add a dash of garlic salt. Bring to boil and simmer for 15 minutes or so. Shirley says, "Spicy, yummy, and very filling!"

ENTREES

Bunless Burger

3 ½ ounce leanest ground beef or chicken breast (or you can use 3 1/2 oz chicken breast or fish)
Mustard (sugar-free)
Onion powder
Garlic, minced or powder
Paprika
Salt & Pepper
Melba toast

Form a burger patty (if using ground meat). Lightly coat meat in mustard. Sprinkle on seasonings and press into place. Crush melba toast (a ziplock bag works great) and coat meat, pressing into place. Fry in pan until cooked thoroughly. Wrap in two large lettuce leaves - romaine works beautifully for this. "Yum yum yum! Pair with some iced tea with stevia and you're set!"

Spinach "Frittata"

This recipe uses eggs. Dr. Simeons states that eggs may be used "if one has an aversion to meat". 1 whole egg + 3 egg whites have approximately the same fat content as 100 grams of chicken breast.

1/2 egg yolk
4 egg whites
1/2 tsp freshly cracked pepper
1/2 tsp basil
dash sea salt
dash garlic powder

Whip egg mixture. Add seasonings. Add fresh spinach. Heat skillet to medium heat. Add quick spray of fat free cooking spray. Add egg mixture. Cook on medium-low heat, covered, until eggs solidify and mixture is thoroughly cooked. Top with more fresh ground pepper, if desired. Can also be cooked in microwave or oven.

Chicken Wraps

3.5 ounces chicken
4 med cabbage leaves

1 garlic clove
3 T. apple cider vinegar
1/4 t onion powder
1/4 T. sea salt
1/4 T. pepper
1 T. fresh ginger
Mix together finely grated ginger, garlic, onion powder, balsamic vinegar, salt, pepper and chicken pieces. Cook until chicken is cooked thoroughly and then add two chopped cabbage leaves, and cook until cabbage is slightly cooked. Take the 2 remaining cabbage leaves and splitting the chicken mixture, place in cabbage leaves and roll into a wrap.

Tilapia
3 1/2 ounces Tilapia
lemon
Pepper
Cayenne Pepper
Heat frying pan until sizzling hot. Squeeze a little lemon on top of tilapia and season with fresh cracked pepper and cayenne. Throw in sizzling hot pan, seasoned side down. Squeeze lemon juice on top side, and add pepper and cayenne. Cook 3 or so minutes. Flip. Cook an additional 2 - 3 or so minutes, until done.

Sweet n Spicy Chicken Wraps
100 grams of chicken
4 cabbage leaves, whole
1 small gala apple, cored and chopped
*2 Tbsp Braggs Liquid Amino Acids (leave out for vlcd stage)
Water
1 Tbsp Tabasco course ground mustard
2 gloves of garlic minced
2 Tbsp organic beef or chicken broth
Pepper to taste
1 tsp onion powder
1 tsp garlic powder
Place chicken in sauté pan with 2 Tbsp Braggs liquid aminos, black pepper, onion powder, and garlic powder. Cook chicken until done, adding water to deglaze pan and keep chicken moist.
While chicken is cooking take another large pan. (I use a 8" pan with high sides so the cabbage leaves lay open and will not tear.) Add water and bring to a boil. Add cabbage leaves, one at a time, and cook until cabbage leaf is

tender and pliable. (I also remove the hard veins of larger leafs). As they are done take out set to side.

Once the chicken is completely cooked remove chicken from the pan, cool, and cut up. Add the minced garlic, 1 Tbsp mustard, and 2 Tbsp broth to pan drippings. Bring to boil and cook your apples in this mixture. Once the apples start cooking down and are tender, return the chopped chicken to the apple mixture. Take your large steamed cabbage leafs and, spooning in the mixture, roll into wraps. Whaley says, this is satisfying, sweet and spicy, and very filling.

Chicken Chili
3.5 oz chicken breast
1 cup chopped tomatoes
1 1/2 Cup of Water
1 Tbsp Apple Cider Vinegar
Onion powder to taste
3 cloves of garlic, minced
1 Tsp Garlic powder
2 Tsp of Chili powder (or to taste) DIVIDED
2 Large Dashes of Hot Sauce DIVIDED
Dash of Cayenne Pepper
Salt and Pepper to taste.

To one saucepan add 1 cup of water, 1 Tbsp Chili powder, 1 tsp Garlic powder, large dash of hot sauce, salt and pepper. Bring to boil and add chicken. Once chicken is done take out to cool and shred.

In another small saucepan, add 1 cup of tomatoes, 1 Tbsp Apple Cider Vinegar, onion powder, minced garlic, 1 Tbsp chili powder, large dash of hot sauce, and salt and pepper to taste, bring to a boil to cook tomatoes down. Adjust seasoning to taste or add water to get to the consistency you desire, once the tomatoes are cooked down. Add the shredded chicken and let simmer. Toni says, this had lots of flavor and the sauce even thickened and was dark brown like chili sauce would be. Serve with a Grissini breadstick.

Citrus Fish
protocol white fish
1 T minced onion
2 T lemon juice
lemon and orange zest to taste
lemon and orange slices
chopped parsley
salt and pepper to taste

stevia to taste

Mix lemon juice with zest and a little stevia. Baste fish with mixture and top with salt, pepper, and lemon and orange slices. Wrap in aluminum foil and bake at 350 degrees for 5-10 minutes or until fish is thoroughly cooked. Serve with lemon and top with parsley.

Delicious Prawns!

3 1/2 ounces prawns
Large handful chopped cabbage
3 T water
1 chopped apple
Mexican spices (onion,garlic,basil,cumin,red pepper,oregeno,jalapeno pepper, cilantro)
Cayenne pepper
salt and pepper

Sprinkle prawns with cayenne pepper, salt, and pepper. Grill quickly in a hot frying pan. Remove from pan. To same pan add water and stir around to get "crusties". Add cabbage and apples, sprinkle with salt and pepper and Mexican seasonings and stir fry until cabbage is a little limp. Transfer to plate and top with prawns.

Balsamic Mustard Crusted Steak

3.5 ounces filet or London broil
1 t. mustard powder
2 t. apple cider vinegar
1/4 t salt
1/2 t freshly ground black pepper
2 garlic cloves (minced)

Mix all seasoning in a mixing bowl. Line a broiler pan with foil and place steak on top. Coat evenly with mustard mixture and let stand 10 minutes. Broil steak to desired doneness. 3 to 4 minutes per side for medium-rare. Let stand 5 minutes before slicing and serving.

Bunless Chicken Burger

3.5 ounces of ground chicken breast
1/4 t. pepper
1/4 t onion salt
1/4 t. onion powder
1t. garlic powder
1/4 t dry mustard
2 Tbsp apple cider vinegar

2 cups spinach

Mix all ingredients into the ground chicken breast and mold into a small patty. Grill or broil and serve with the spinach and balsamic vinaigrette.

Chilean Sea Bass

3.5 ounces of sea bass fillets
2 cloves garlic, minced
1/2 of lemon
1/2 t. salt
1/2 t. lemon pepper
2 T. finely chopped cilantro
1/2 t. paprika

Arrange Sea bass fillets in a single layer on foil-lined broiler pan. Spread garlic and cilantro on and around fish. Squeeze lemon juice on fillets, sprinkle salt and lemon pepper to taste, and add paprika for color. Cover with foil and crimp edges to form a seal.

Bake at 450 for 20 minutes

Spicy Chicken & Cabbage Soup with Chicken & Cabbage Stir-fry

3 * oz chicken breast
2 cups cabbage, shredded
salt, pepper, bay leaf, dried parsley, cayenne pepper

Place chicken breast portion in medium saucepan filled halfway with water. Add plenty of fresh ground black pepper, dash of sea salt; bay leaf; dried parsley. Bring to boil, then simmer, until chicken is cooked. Pull chicken from broth and finely shred it. Add 2 Tbsp of the chicken broth, dash of cayenne pepper, and fresh ground pepper. Mix together. Toss 1/2 of the cabbage mixture and * of the shredded chicken mixture into broth and simmer, another five or so minutes. Heat frying pan until very hot. Toss remaining cabbage/chicken mixture into frying pan, and cook until crisp/tender. Pour soup into bowl and place cabbage onto plate. Thelma says this is a delicious meal with plenty of *ZING* ... filling and very satisfying!

Citrus Halibut

3.5 ounces halibut
2 T. fresh lemon juice
1 garlic clove, minced
1/2 teaspoon dried thyme
1/2 teaspoon dried dill

1/4 t pepper
1/4 t salt
1/2 citrus dressing

Mix together lemon juice, lime juice, garlic, thyme, and salt and pepper to taste. Place in a shallow dish, drizzle with citrus dressing mixture, turn to coat and marinate at room temperature for 10 minutes. Heat grill pan or grill over medium heat. Cook for 3 to 4 minutes per side.

Curry Chicken and Spinach

3.5 ounces chicken
2 cups spinach
2 t. onion powder
1 garlic clove (minced)
1/2 cup chicken broth
1/4 t salt
1/4 t pepper
1 lemon
1 T. curry powder

Mix chicken and all seasonings and 1/2 the lemon and cook chicken through. Throw the spinach in for 1 minute and serve in a bowl and squeeze the other 1/2 of the lemon.

Ginger Steamed White Fish

3.5 ounces white fish
2T. fresh grated ginger
1/4 cup apple cider vinegar
2 drops liquid stevia
1/4 t. salt
1/4 t. pepper
1 lemon wedge

Finely grate 1 T of fresh ginger in small skillet. Add the balsamic vinegar and cover with water to reach 2 inches and bring to a simmer. Season red snapper with grated ginger, lemon, salt and pepper. Place in steamer and cook for about 10 minutes.

Lemon Garlic Chard

2c. roughly chopped Swiss chard
1 large or 2 small garlic cloves
4 T. water
Fresh lemon juice
Sea salt

Pepper

Put 1 T. water in non stick pan sauté garlic until tender and set aside. Pour remaining water into pan and add chard. Cook over medium heat for about 5 minutes, tossing occasionally. Drain off excess juice and return to pan adding in sautéed garlic. Before serving, give a squirt of lemon juice and a shake of salt and pepper.

Lemon Tilapia

3.5 ounces tilapia or any white fish
1 lemon slice
1 garlic clove (minced)
1/4 T. sea salt
1/4 T. black pepper
1/2 t. dry dill
1/2 cup water

Mix together lemon juice, lime juice, garlic, salt, pepper, and dill. Marinate fish in seasonings for 10 minutes and place in non-stick pan with water and cover and steam for 10 minutes.

LisaBE's Breaded Pan-Seared Tilapia

3.5 oz tilapia
1 Melba toast
Garlic salt
Parsley
Dill
Salt & Pepper
2 -3 Tbsp sugar-free tomato sauce

Place melba toast in baggie and smashed it with a wooden spoon. Lisa says: a very satisfying act. Add to bag the garlic salt, parsley, dill, salt and pepper. Coat tilapia with sugar-free tomato sauce. Rub in crumb mixture. Spray a *quick* shot of fat-free cooking spray into non-stick pan. Heat pan. Add breaded fish. Add just a little water, cover with lid, and cook until done, about 3 - 4 minutes, each side.

Cider vinegar chicken - vlcd

3.5 oz chicken, sprinkle both sides liberally with garlic salt & pepper,
cover with about 1/4-1/2 cup of cider vinegar
bake on 350degrees for 25-30 min (or until juices run clear)
Optional: add a few red chili pepper flakes to vinegar for a bit of heat

Have it on it's own, or chop and add to bed of lettuce.

Lemon Zest Crab Cakes
3.5 ounces crab
1 garlic clove (minced)
1 T. onion powder
1/2 t. lemon zest
1/4 t salt
1/4 t. pepper
1 t. dry mustard
2 lemon wedges
1 T. parsley
1 t. lemon zest
Mix everything together and put into 2 small patties. Place in a baking dish
and bake for 15 minutes and place on serving dish.

Marinated London Broil Steak & Salsa
3.5 ounces London broil
1/3 cup apple cider vinegar
2T. dried Oregano
3T. garlic powder
1/4 t salt
1/4 t pepper
2 cups diced tomatoes
Marinate London broil with all seasons for 1 hour. Season diced tomatoes and
place 1/2 in the middle of the plate. Broil or grill steak to your temperature.
Place on top of salsa and add the remainder salsa.

Mock Egg Roll
3.5 ounces of chicken breast OR lean steak, cut into strips OR shrimp OR lean
ground chicken breast or beef
2-3 big cabbage leaves
1c. shredded cabbage

1/8 t. onion salt
1/8 t. garlic powder
1/8 Asian spices
2 - 3 drops liquid stevia
Cook meat of your choice. Steam big cabbage leaves for 5 minutes. Move leaves over to side of steamer to make room for shredded cabbage. Steam both for 5 minutes. Remove shredded cabbage to a mixing bowl. Add chopped meat and spices. Mix and then wrap in a big cabbage leaf.

Oven Chicken Salad with Vinaigrette Dressing
1 chicken breast portion
1/2 t. cayenne pepper (optional)
1/4 t. onion powder
1/4 t. salt
1/4 t. pepper
1/4 t. garlic powder
1/2 t. poultry season
2 cups spinach or lettuce
Cut chicken into cubes. Toss in seasonings. Bake at 325 until chicken is cooked through. Top spinach or lettuce with chicken.

Rosemary Fish & Lemon Garlic Chard
3.5 ounces of tilapia
Italian Herb Seasoning
1 t. Rosemary grinded
1 t. Ground pepper
1 t. Sea Salt
2 slices of fresh lemon juice
1 t. garlic salt
Sprinkle both sides of fish with spices. Place fish on a nonstick frying pan with 1/3 cup of water and lemon juice. Place a lid on the pan to keep the steam within the pan. Cook for 3 to 4 min. Fish is done when flakes easily with a fork. Serve with your favorite protocol vegetable, like steamed spinach.

Spicy Cajun Shrimp
3.5 ounces shrimp
1 lemon
1/2 dry mustard
1 t. pepper flakes
2 garlic clove (minced)
1/4 salts

1/4 pepper
1/2 cup water
Mix together lemon juice, dry mustard, cayenne, garlic, salt, pepper and shrimp. Fill a non-stick frying pan with water and place shrimp and cover with lid for10 minutes.

Spicy Taco Salad
2 cups Romaine Lettuce
3.5 ounces London broil or filet
1/4 t. garlic salt
1/4 t. chili seasoning
Prepare the beef on the grill. Crumble beef and mix in garlic, salt, and chili seasoning. Top lettuce with ground beef mixture. Serve with Vinaigrette Dressing on the side.

DESSERTS

Apple Cobbler
1 sliced apple
1/8 t. cinnamon
2- 3 drops liquid stevia
Toss the above ingredients and arrange on oven safe dish. Then add topping.
Topping:
1 melba toast
Sprinkle apples with the crumbled melba toast, cinnamon, and stevia.
Microwave for 2 minutes on high.

Apple Sauce
Bake apple. Peel off skin. Mash. Add cinnamon and 2 -3 drops of liquid stevia. Mix all together and serve.

Baked Apple
Any apple you like
2 - 3 drops liquid stevia
1 T. cinnamon
1 T. cinnamon
1 t. water

Remove apple core but keep apple whole. Place apple in oven-proof dish. Sprinkle inside with stevia and cinnamon. Sprinkle on water. Bake at 350 for 30 - 45 minutes. Enjoy with a cup of hot tea.

Jamaican Grapefruit
1/2 grapefruit
Cinnamon
2 - 3 drops liquid stevia, or to taste
Using a serrated edge knife, cut grapefruit in half as normally would and place on an oven safe dish and bake for 2 minutes. Cut around center core, rind, and partitions. Sprinkle with cinnamon and stevia.

Strawberry Flower
4 large strawberries or 6 small
1 T. cinnamon
2 - 3 drops liquid stevia, or to taste
Slice strawberries and place on a plate shaped like a flower. Mix cinnamon and stevia and sprinkle over the strawberries.

MAINTENANCE RECIPES

BEVERAGES

Strawberry Maintenance-Rita
Crushed Ice
3 large frozen strawberries
2 shots Jose' Cuervo
2 1/2 shots lime juice
1 shot lemon juice
Stevia to taste
Blend and Enjoy! "For anyone who has a special occasion during Maintenance, here is an "adult beverage" you may safely enjoy, in moderation."

SkinnyRita
Tonic Water
Tequila

1/2 lime

Pour tonic water over ice; add tequila; cut 1/2 lime in half again, squeeze both sections over glass; add the lime segments to the glass and enjoy! "You may enjoy an occasional alcohol beverage but we recommend you wait until after your critical first week of Maintenance. Cheers!"

DRESSINGS, BROTHS, SAUCES

Marinara ~ Maintenance
tomato sauce (sugar free)
olive oil
fresh (or dried) grated onion
garlic powder
basil
salt
pepper

Combine all ingredients. If you want even CHUNKIER sauce add bell peppers and mushrooms .

Homemade (SF) Mayo
3 large Eggs
3 Tbsp vinegar
1 tsp sea salt
3/4 tsp dry mustard
1 pack of stevia (optional)
3 cup oil
juice of one lemon

**you could add some fresh herbs at this point if you like)

In a blender put eggs, vinegar, sea salt and dry mustard and blend until mixed. With the blender still running, slowly pour 1 1/2 cups oil into blender, add lemon juice and blend for about 1 min, slowly add the rest of the oil (1 1/2 c.) and
blend till it has consistency and color of Mayo.

Keep Refrigerated.

This recipe makes approximately one jar of Mayo, if you want or need less just adjust the recipe.

Coconut Mayonnaise

Ingredients:
1 egg
1 Tbsp apple cider vinegar
* Tbsp prepared mustard
* tsp paprika
* tsp salt
1* C melted coconut oil

Directions:
Blend the first 5 ingredients plus 1* C of the coconut oil for 60 seconds. While machine is running, pour in the remaining oil very slowly in a fine, steady stream.

Each Tbsp of the mayo will have about 1* Tbsp coconut oil. If you have been using coconut oil, you will know that this will harden in the fridge; just let it sit at room temperature half an hour or so to soften. Use within several days. The texture is best when freshly made.

APPETIZERS, SIDES, SALADS AND SOUPS

Fauxtato Salad
1 cauliflower cut into florets
1/2 cup sliced scallions
3 celery ribs
1/2 green bell pepper
1/4 cup parsley
salt and pepper

dressing
2 tsp dry mustard (Coleman's)
2 tbsp apple cider vinegar
1 cup mayo

3 hard boiled eggs chopped

1/2 -1 tsp celery seeds
paprika for garnish

Steam cauliflower florets until tender and set aside. Put scallions, celery, bell pepper, parsley, salt and pepper in a bowl. When cauliflower is cool, add it to other vegetables. Mix in enough dressing to just coat the vegetables. Stir in eggs and celery seeds. Sprinkle paprika on top. Cover with plastic wrap and set in fridge for 2 hours.

Chicken Lemon "Rice" Soup ~Maintenance
2 cups chicken broth (sugar-free)
2 cups water
2 - 3 tsp poultry seasoning (sugar-free)
4 servings chicken (thawed or frozen)
1 head cauliflower, florets removed in large pieces
2 stalks celery (cut into large pieces) or 1 tsp celery salt
juice and zest of 2 lemons
Put all ingredients in crock pot. Add water if the cauliflower is not covered. Cook on low 4 - 6 hours (depending on whether your chicken was frozen, or not.). Remove cauliflower with slotted spoon. Put in blender, filling only halfway. Add 1 cup of broth. Vent so this doesn't explode when blending. Blend - longer for creamy, shorter for chunky. Add creamed cauliflower back to soup, and repeat with more cauliflower florets. Remove chicken and shred. You can add a squeeze of lemon or lemon zest, if desired. Carrie says, "It's so yummy! If you leave the cauliflower a little chunky, it almost feels like you're eating rice! Mmmm!"

Green Layered Salad ~Maintenance ~ enough for a group gathering and a big crowd-pleaser!
1 medium head lettuce
1/2 cup chopped green onion
1 cup chopped celery
8 oz sliced water chestnuts
1 10 oz can green peas (no sugar added)
2 cups sugar-free mayo (Best Foods or Hellmann's are good choices)
Stevia to taste
1/2 cup grated Parmesan
1/4 tsp garlic salt
1/4 tsp fresh cracked pepper
1/4 tsp onion flakes

3 grated hard boiled eggs
1 lb cooked and crumbled crisp bacon
tomato wedges
dried parsley
1st layer: Shred lettuce in large bowl. Add onion, celery, chestnuts, and peas - mix together - spread on bottom of oblong serving dish.
2nd layer: Mix mayo, stevia, Parmesan, seasonings. Spread on top of 1st layer. Sprinkle with egg and bacon. Top with tomato wedges and parsley.
Audrey says: if you are close to your 2 lb limit push the water chestnuts and peas to the side, or leave them out altogether, as they are *caution* veggies.

Au Gratin Cauliflower ~Maintenance
2 cups cauliflower, cooked and finely chopped
1/2 cup sour cream
1 cup grated cheese, your favorite
2 Tbsp finely chopped or dried basil
1/4 tsp garlic powder
salt
pepper
Mix cooked and finely chopped cauliflower with sour cream, grated cheese, finely chopped or dried basil, garlic, salt, and freshly ground pepper. Spread and press into casserole dish. Bake at 350 degrees until golden brown and slightly crusted edges. Audrey says, this was so darned good I felt like I was eating something very bad!

Stuffed Jalapenos/Guero Peppers ~Maintenance
1 cup cream cheese
2 cups shredded mozzarella cheese
Mix as well as you can. Cut up half a package of turkey bacon or turkey sausage and brown in a pan. Add to cheese mixture. Fill the peppers with a Tbsp. of mixture and place in oven @ 450 degrees for 15-20 minutes, or until cheese is all the way melted and a little browned. Cathy says, This makes a very large batch. SO good! Eat with caution though.

Oopsie Rolls ~ Maintenance
3 large eggs
pinch of cream of tartar (1/8 tsp)
3 ounces cream cheese (do not soften)
Preheat oven to 300 degrees. Separate the eggs. Beat egg whites and cream of tartar until VERY STIFF - peaks should hold. Then mix the egg yolks with the cream cheese - it should have a "cottage cheese" consistency. Using a

large spatula gradually fold the egg yolk mixture into the white mixture, being careful not to break down the whites. Spray a cookie sheet with non-stick spray and carefully scoop the mixture onto the sheet, making six mounds. Flatten each mound softly. Bake 30 minutes. Let cool on sheet for a few minutes, then transfer to rack to cool. Store in a paper bag. May be frozen. Thelma says: These are DELICIOUS as hamburger buns, or with egg, or a sandwich! I added a blend of spices to the yolk mixture followed by a sprinkling on top of the mounds for the hamburger buns - yummy! You may add stevia to the yolk mixture for a sweeter roll.

Cauliflower Pizza Bread ~ Maintenance
1 cup cooked, riced cauliflower *see instructions below
1 egg
1 cup mozzarella cheese
1/2 tsp fennel
1 tsp oregano
2 tsp parsley
Preheat oven to 450 degrees Fahrenheit. Spray a cookie sheet with non-stick spray. In medium bowl, combine cauliflower, egg and mozzarella. Press evenly on the pan. Sprinkle evenly with fennel, oregano and parsley. Bake at 450 degrees for 12-15 minutes (15-20 minutes if you double the recipe). Remove the pan from the oven. Slice into strips. Dunk in heated Marinara Sauce (recipe above). Thelma says: Delicious! A GREAT "dipping bread" !
*You may use frozen cauliflower prepared according to package directions. Cook and slightly cool, shred with cheese grater, measure for recipe - don't pack down measuring cup - just fill to top.

Yummy "Eggplant Parmesan Pizza Circles" ~ Maintenance
1/2 eggplant, sliced into circles
1 egg, beaten, + 1 Tbsp milk, half-n-half, or whipping cream
Italian Seasoning (sugar-free)
Basil flakes
Parsley flakes
Garlic powder
Cayenne pepper
Pepper flakes
1/4 cup shredded Parmesan cheese, divided in half
Place a rack on cookie sheet and spray with fat free cooking spray. Slice eggplant into circles. Combine egg, seasonings (to taste), and 1/2 the cheese. Mix together. Dip each eggplant circle into the egg mixture, coating thoroughly. Place eggplant on rack. Top with remaining Parmesan cheese.

Bake in preheated oven at 400 degrees until golden brown. Serve on platter with heated Marinara Sauce (recipe in Sauces, above.) Thelma says, This was such a great "starchy" tasting treat ~ a cross between pizza and eggplant marinara!

Favorite Cauliflower Faux Tater Tots
1 12 ounce bag frozen cauliflower
1/3 cup grated Parmesan Cheese
salt, pepper, onion powder (to taste)
Cook cauliflower, covered, in microwave for 6 minutes. Pour off water and let stand until cool. Grate cauliflower in a food processor or with grater. Form cauliflower into 1.5* balls, squeezing and working any excess water as you do so. Drop into Parmesan. Form into tots by flattening the tops. If the mixture is still too moist and falls apart, work a little of the Parmesan into the tot, and then roll the formed tots into the Parmesan once again to coat. Place tots on a greased cookie sheet and freeze for 30 minutes prior to baking to help tots hold their shape. At this point it's good to note that you can freeze them longer or make these ahead of time. Simply place in a freezer bag after the initial chilling period and store for up to a month. Bake in preheated 400 degree oven for 10 minutes, rotating once for even browning. Optional: serve topped with Yer Darned Tootin* Chile & American Cheese

Yer Darned Tootin* Chili

1 lb ground beef
1 can Rotel
* cup minced purple onion
2 cloves garlic
1 Tbsp cocoa powder
1 Tbsp cumin
1 Tbsp chili powder
1 tsp salt
1 tsp oregano
Brown ground beef. Add Rotel, with liquid, and chop in with ground beef. Add remaining ingredients. Bring to boil, then simmer for 20 minutes, uncovered, stirring occasionally.

American Cheese Sauce
2 Tbsp butter
2 Tbsp heavy cream

4 oz American Cheese
* tsp salt
Melt butter in small pan over medium heat. Add cream and water. Add cheese and salt. Cook, stirring occasionally, until cheese has melted, about 5 - 10 minutes. Add 1 Tbsp water if thinner consistency is desired.

Zucchini Doritos-style chips

1 large zucchini, shredded
2 eggs
2 cups cheese

Preheat oven to 450 degrees F.
Grease 2 cookie sheets.

Cut ends from zucchini. Shred. Mix with egg and cheese. Make 6-8* circles on greased cookie sheet(s). Bake at 450 degrees for 12 minutes. Loosen and flip the circles. Bake for another 5 minutes at 450 degrees.

With a pizza cutter, cut rounds into triangles (about 6 per round).

Let cool on a rack for 6-8 hours in a cool oven. To store, keep loosely in a bag or a plastic container in the refrigerator or on the counter. Best used within a week of preparation.

After chips have dried substantially, in a plastic container toss with popcorn seasoning for desired flavor.
Makes 36 chips.

Nutritional Information:(Per 12 chips, 1/3 of recipe): Calories: 151, Carbohydrates: 1g, Fiber: 0g, Net Carbohydrates: 1 g, Protein: 10 g, Fat: 13 g

Cauliflower Doritos-style chips

1 16 ounce bag of cauliflower, shredded, chopped or riced
3 eggs

3 cups cheese

Preheat oven to 450 degrees F.
Grease 2 cookie sheets.

Cook or thaw frozen cauliflower. Shred, rice or chop. Mix with egg and cheese. Using 1/4 cup scoop, make 12 6-8* circles on greased cookie sheet(s). Bake at 450 degrees for 12 minutes. Loosen and flip the circles. Bake for another 5 minutes at 450 degrees.

With a pizza cutter, cut rounds into triangles (about 6 per round).

Let cool on a rack for 6-8 hours in a cool oven. To store, keep loosely in a bag or a plastic container in the refrigerator or on the counter. Best used within a week of preparation.

Notes: Recipes can be halved for less chips.
Store on rack until crisp and then in an open container to prevent moisture.

After chips have dried substantially, in a plastic container toss with popcorn seasoning for desired flavor.

Makes 72 chips.
Nutritional Information (Per 12 chips, 1/6 of recipe): Calories: 239, Carbohydrates: 4g, Fiber: 1.5g, Net Carbohydrates: 2.5 g, Protein: 15 g, Fat: 20 g

Spinach Omelet in a bag
eggs
spinach
sm ziplock FREEZER expandable bottom bags

in a large pan boil water.
chop fresh spinach, whisk 1 whole egg, 3 egg whites /combine in bag
cook in boiled water, cover pot for 15-20 mins on high!!!

(for spice sprinkle Tabasco sauce)
as for MAINTENANCE= add fresh mushrooms, tomatoes & jalapenos

Pesto Cream Cheese Stuffed Cherry Tomatoes

Ingredients

- Healthy size handful of basil leaves (the whole container if using one of those plastic 0.75 oz fresh herb packs)
- clove of garlic (a really bitter piece of garlic could ruin everything so be careful!)
- 1/4 cup pine nuts
- 1/4 grated parmesan
- 1 6-8 oz size pkg low fat (not reduced fat) cream cheese. I used the Philly with 1/3 less fat.
- 1 pint cherry tomatoes (the slightly bigger ones are ideal)

How to make it

- Throw everything but the tomatoes into the food processor and process until it is paste like.
- Hollow out the cherry tomatoes
- Put the pesto cream cheese in a baggie, cut the tip off of one of the bottom corners of the bag to create a 'pastry' type bag, and pipe the cheese mixture into the tomatoes
- Sprinkle chopped basil on top for garnish if desired.
- This also works well as an appetizer if you spread the pesto cheese on a crostini and then top it with a tomato slice. The cream cheese pesto alone is dip worthy with veggies, pita chips, crackers, anything. Tasty.
- Cook down the garlic for 1 min or so before you add it to the mix if you don't want the intensity of raw garlic flavor.
- Also, if you make it ahead be aware that the garlic flavor will intensify over time.

Mixed Berry Muffins
These yummy muffins are great for dessert or a snack

2 cups almond flour
Stevia equivalent to 2 T sugar
1 t baking powder
1 cup butter melted and cooled slightly
1 cup cream
4 eggs

1 t orange or lemon extract
1 t vanilla extract
1 cup mixed berries of choice

Tip: freeze the berries first and toss them in a tablespoon of the almond flour. It will keep the berries suspended in the batter during cooking.

1 t xanthan gum (optional, but makes for a much nicer finished product)
Line 2 muffin pans with muffin cups. Preheat oven to 350 degrees.

In a medium bowl, mix the wet ingredients. In larger bowl, mix the dry ingredients (except berries). Mix only until combined, do not beat. Mix in berries and divide between muffin cups.

Bake for 20-25 minutes until golden brown and firm to the touch. Leave on cooling rack for 15-20 minutes.

Coconut Flour Pancakes...

2 eggs
2 tablespoons coconut oil or butter, melted
2 tablespoons coconut milk or whole milk (I used 2%)
1 teaspoon sugar (I used 1/4 tsp stevia granules)
1/8 teaspoon salt
2 tablespoons sifted coconut flour (I didn't sift)
1/8 teaspoon baking powder

Directions: Blend together eggs, oil, coconut milk, sugar or substitute, and salt. Combine coconut flour and baking powder and thoroughly mix into batter. Heat 1 tablespoon of coconut oil in a skillet. Spoon batter onto hot skillet making pancakes about 2 1/2 to 3 inches in diameter. Batter will be thick but will flatten out when cooking. Makes about 8 small pancakes.

This is enough for one serving, really. Texture is similar to crepes but thicker. I served with hot sliced pears!

Guilt-free Waffles

2 large eggs

1/4* C Ricotta cheese
1/4* tsp cinnamon
1/8 tsp. Nutmeg (optional)
1/2* tsp. Baking powder
1-2 packages Stevia
Preheat waffle iron. (Can also be made into pancakes.) Beat eggs with electric mixer or whisk to make them light and fluffy. Add all other ingredients and beat until smooth. Spray waffle maker with MCT oil or other cooking spray. Pour in batter and cook as usual for waffles.

Cauli-Tater Salad

1-16 ounce bag cauliflower, chopped
1* cup red, green, yellow bell peppers (each), chopped
1/2 red onion, chopped
1 kosher baby dill pickles, chopped
1 Tomato, chopped
1 hard-boiled eggs, peeled and chopped
1 Tbsp mustard
1/2 cup mayonnaise (nsa)
1/2 cup sour cream (read label for sugar)
1 tbsp ACV
1/2 tsp Celtic salt
1/4* tsp pepper
garlic powder for taste
dash of sweetener of choice
nsa ham or turkey (optional)

Cook cauliflower but not too soft, drain and rinse with cold water. Chop cauliflower and all other veggies and put in medium size bowl. Make dressing out of mayo, mustard, sour cream, ACV and seasonings and add to bowl with cauliflower.
Mix well and Enjoy =)

Parmesan chips
 recipe from Michelle

You can use Parmesan or other super hard cheeses.

Preheat oven to 350.

Place small piles of grated Parmesan (the grated kind works best, avoid the powdery stuff) on a parchment lined cookie sheet.... See More

Flatten them a bit.

You can sprinkle with a little seasoning is you like. Garlic, basil, Italian seasonings.

Bake until golden brown.

You can make larger crackers, and when they are still soft from the oven shape them into "baskets" for salads etc...

Zucchini Mash
great substitute for mashed potatoes

yield: Makes 4 to 6 servings

1 medium green bell pepper, finely chopped (1 cup)
2 tablespoons extra-virgin olive oil
2 tablespoons unsalted butter
1 large garlic clove, finely chopped
6 medium zucchini (1 3/4 pounds), halved lengthwise, then thinly sliced crosswise
1/2 cup water
3/4 teaspoon salt
1/2 teaspoon black pepper
1/3 cup chopped scallion greens

Cook bell pepper in oil and 1 tablespoon butter in a wide 4-quart heavy pot over moderately low heat, stirring occasionally, until softened, 4 to 6 minutes. Add garlic and cook, stirring, 1 minute. Add zucchini, water, salt, and pepper and bring to a boil over moderately high heat, then cook at a brisk simmer, covered, 6 minutes. Remove lid and simmer until most of liquid is evaporated and zucchini is soft, about 6 minutes.

Coarsely mash zucchini with a potato masher and add scallion greens and remaining tablespoon butter, stirring, until butter is incorporated

great substitute for mashed potatoes
yield: Makes 4 to 6 servings
active time: 15 min
total time: 35 min
Toss aside the mashed potatoes and welcome this appealing alternative, a spirited mix of zucchini, tender sautéed bell pepper, and refreshing scallions.

1 medium green bell pepper, finely chopped (1 cup)
2 tablespoons extra-virgin olive oil
2 tablespoons unsalted butter
1 large garlic clove, finely chopped
6 medium zucchini (1 3/4 pounds), halved lengthwise, then thinly sliced crosswise
1/2 cup water
3/4 teaspoon salt
1/2 teaspoon black pepper
1/3 cup chopped scallion greens

Preparation Cook bell pepper in oil and 1 tablespoon butter in a wide 4-quart heavy pot over moderately low heat, stirring occasionally, until softened, 4 to 6 minutes. Add garlic and cook, stirring, 1 minute. Add zucchini, water, salt, and pepper and bring to a boil over moderately high heat, then cook at a brisk simmer, covered, 6 minutes. Remove lid and simmer until most of liquid is evaporated and zucchini is soft, about 6 minutes.

Coarsely mash zucchini with a potato masher and add scallion greens and remaining tablespoon butter, stirring, until butter is incorporated

Gluten Free Pizza using the Gluten Free Crust
Makes 2-4 servings

2 cups whole milk organic mozzarella cheese, shredded
2 large organic eggs
2 tablespoons flax meal
2 tablespoons coconut flour
1* teaspoon baking powder

Preparation:
Preheat oven to 350 degrees F. Cut 2 pieces of parchment paper out for baking sheet. Mix cheese, eggs, flax, coconut flour, and baking powder together until

a sticky wet dough is formed. Spread with a spatula to * inch thickness on a baking sheet lined with one piece of parchment paper.

Bake for 30 minutes in preheated oven. Halfway through the baking process, flip crust over by sliding it off the baking sheet with the parchment paper, placing the second piece on the sheet, and turning the crust over unto the new sheet and peeling the old paper off. Return to oven until done baking.

Remove from oven, slide off of parchment paper, and flip over again for cooling. Once crust is cooled, top with sauce, pre-cooked veggies or meats, and cheese. Set crust with toppings under the broiler on high for a minute or two until cheese is melted and bubbly.

Slice and serve.
Recipe submitted by Lauren, Fort Myers, FLTropical Traditions

Low-Carb Pancakes - Almond Meal
Almond meal differs a bit from one batch to the other, so you may have to adjust the amount of liquid to get the thickness you want.

Ingredients:

* 1 cup almond flour
* 2 eggs
* 1/4 cup water (for puffier pancakes, you can use sparkling water)
* 2 T oil
* 1/4 teaspoon salt
* 1 T sweetener

Preparation:
Mix ingredients together and cook as you would other pancakes. I like to use a nonstick pan with a little oil. The only real difference is that they won't "bubble" on top the same way as regular pancakes. Flip them when the underside is brown.

Serve with sugar-free maple syrup, Easy Three Berry Syrup, strawberry topping, or other low carb topping.

Yield: Six 4-inch pancakes

Nutritional Information: Each pancake has 1 gram effective carbohydrate, plus 2 grams of fiber, 6 grams of protein, and 155 calories.

ENTREES

Coconut Flour Pancakes
2 eggs
2 Tbsp coconut oil or butter, melted
2 Tbsp coconut or regular milk
Stevia (1/4 tsp stevia granules or liquid stevia to taste)
1/8 tsp salt
2 Tbsp coconut flour
1/8 tsp baking powder (Note: sub pinch of baking soda + pinch of cream of tartar for "starch-free" recipe)
Blend together eggs, oil, coconut milk, stevia, and salt. Combine coconut flour and baking powder and thoroughly mix into batter. Heat 1 tbsp. coconut oil in skillet. Spoon batter onto hot skillet, making pancakes about 2 1/2 - 3 inches in diameter. Batter will be thick but will flatten out when cooking. Makes about 8 small pancakes. "This is enough for one serving, really. Texture is similar to crepes, but thicker. I served with hot sliced pears!"

Cream Cheese Pancakes
1 8 oz softened cream cheese
4 eggs separated
1/2 to 1 tsp stevia granules, or 1-2 packets
1/2 to 1 tsp Cinnamon (to taste)
butter for griddle

1. Beat egg white till stiff with peaks
2. with a hand mixer: Beat egg yolks & cream cheese until creamy
add in stevia & cinnamon
3. "FOLD" egg white gently into egg yolks
4. on a medium to med. high griddle/pan melt butter (1 Tbs.)
5. Put pancakes size dollops in pan and cook until edges are brown and the bubbles pop and stay open.
6. Flip and do the same

This batch made 9 nice sized pancakes! Serve with Strawberries & sugar-free whipped cream, (or any fresh fruit), or sugar free syrup. Trish says, "DELICIOUS!!"

Parmesan 'Fried' Chicken ~ Maintenance

2 lbs chicken breasts (cut into 6 oz servings, serves 5)
1 cup parmesan cheese (use the real stuff, not the imitation)
1/2 cup almond flour
2 Tbsp Italian Seasoning
1 egg
3 Tbsp olive oil

Preheat oven to 350 degrees. Mix all dry ingredients. Make egg wash out of egg and water. Dip chicken breast pieces into egg wash and then into Parmesan mixture, set aside. Heat large non-stick pan with olive oil on medium high. Once pan and oil are thoroughly heated place chicken pieces in pan and brown on both sides. After browned, place in a baking dish that you've sprayed with a tiny bit of cooking spray. Bake at 350 degrees for about 20 - 25 minutes, until cooked through. Enjoy the yummy! Brandi says, "I actually created this recipe before starting hCG, when I was trying to cut out white flour ... and then I realized that it worked for P3 (Maintenance) as well."

Baked Almond Chicken

This is a delicious and filling dinner entrée.

1 teaspoon celery salt
1 teaspoon paprika
1/2* teaspoon seasoned salt
1 teaspoon curry powder
1/4* teaspoon pepper
6 boneless, skinless chicken breasts
1 cup whipping cream
1/4* teaspoon almond extract
1/2* cup sliced or slivered toasted almonds

Arrange chicken in a greased shallow 3 qt. baking dish.

Mix seasonings into cream.

Pour the seasoned cream around chicken.

Bake uncovered, at 350 degrees for 45 minutes.

Top with almonds.

Bake uncovered, for 5-8 minutes or until golden brown.

Chicken or Pork with Creamy White Sauce ~ Maintenance

4 boneless skinless chicken breast halves or boneless pork chops
2 Tbsp butter
1/2 c white cooking wine (or sugar-free chicken broth)
1/2 c heavy whipping cream (or half-n-half, or milk)
1 Tbsp minced fresh rosemary (or fresh basil)
1 cup of sliced mushrooms
Spray large skillet with fat free cooking spray. Cook chicken or pork chops over medium heat. Remove and keep warm. Add wine to the pan and cook over medium-low heat, stirring to loosen browned bits from pan. Add cream and bring to boil. Reduce heat and stir until slightly thickened. Add rosemary and remaining butter until blended. Add mushrooms and return meat to pan. Serve sauce with chicken

Cauliflower Pizza ~Maintenance

1 cup cooked, riced cauliflower *see instructions below
1 egg
1 cup mozzarella cheese
1/2 tsp fennel
1 tsp oregano
2 tsp parsley
sugar-free pizza or Alfredo sauce
toppings (make sure meats are cooked)
mozzarella cheese

Preheat oven to 450 degrees Fahrenheit. Spray a cookie sheet with non-stick spray. In medium bowl, combine cauliflower, egg and mozzarella. Press evenly on the pan. Sprinkle evenly with fennel, oregano and parsley. Bake at 450 degrees for 12-15 minutes (15-20 minutes if you double the recipe). Remove the pan from the oven. To the crust, add sauce, then toppings and cheese. Place under broiler at high heat just until cheese is melted.
Additional Tips
*You may use frozen cauliflower prepared according to package directions. Cook and slightly cool, shred with cheese grater, measure for recipe - don't pack down measuring cup - just fill to top.
Thelma says: Delicious! This would also make a GREAT "dipping bread" baked with just cheese, then sliced up and dipped in pizza or Alfredo sauce!

Meaty Eggplant Parmesan

Serving Size: 8
Ingredients
1 pound extra-lean ground beef
4 tablespoon olive oil ; divided
2 tablespoon diced or grated white onion
Garlic ; to taste
1 tablespoon freshly-ground black pepper
2 large eggplants - (about 3 lbs)
3 large eggs ; lightly beaten
1 cup vital wheat gluten flour
1/2 cup finely-crushed pork rinds
1 cup grated Parmesan cheese ; divided
16 ounces low-carb no-sugar Italian sauce (Classico Italian Sauce works well)
Shredded mozzarella cheese

Instructions
Peel eggplant; cut into 1/4-inch slices. Place in a deep bowl and cover with cool water. Allow to sit for 5 minutes, then drain, rinse, and cover again with fresh water. Set aside for 10 minutes. (You'll notice the water turning greenish purple at first and will finally run clear.)

Meanwhile brown ground beef in skillet with 2 tablespoons olive oil, black pepper, grated onion and garlic. Remove from skillet and set aside.

In a medium bowl combine vital wheat gluten flour, crushed pork rinds, and 1/4 cup parmesan cheese. Sift to mix well.

66

Preheat oven to 400 degrees. Dry eggplant slices completely on paper towels. Prepare 2 cookie sheets with a fine coating of remaining olive oil.

Dip each slice into beaten egg to coat, then into flour mixture. Place each on cookie sheet and bake for 10 to 15 minutes. Turn eggplant slices, and bake an additional 7 minutes. Repeat as necessary until all eggplant slices are baked and browned.

Reduce oven to 350 degrees. Lightly grease (with oil or Pam) a 13- by 9- by 2-inch baking dish. Cover bottom with ground beef mixture. Then layer browned eggplant slices across top; add sauce and parmesan cheese; repeat layers until all eggplant and sauce is used.

Cover with a layer of shredded mozzarella cheese and bake at 350 degrees for 30 minutes or until thoroughly heated and top cheese is melted, bubbly, and beginning to brown.

Allow to sit for 10 minutes before serving. Enjoy!

This recipe yields 8 servings; 7 carb grams per serving (assuming Classico Sauce - adjust count for the sauce used if needed.)

**According to Linda Prinster, vital wheat gluten is allowed on P3, not even a cautionary food on her list. The recipe might be worth a try if you really want some Italian food.

Calzones!

1 batch dough:
1 large eggplant, shredded (or zucchini)
1 egg
1 cup shredded mozzarella
Pizza sauce (I use Contadina Thick and Zesty Tomato sauce with spices)
Toppings (turkey pepperoni, chicken sausage, olives, mushrooms)
Shredded cheese (GOAT cheese anyone!?)

Peel the outside off and cut up eggplant into long lasagna noodle-shaped strips. Place on a sprayed cookie sheet, sprinkle with salt and bake for 15 minutes (to get some moisture out). Preheat oven to 450 degrees F. In a food processor, blend eggplant, egg and cheese. Grease a cookie sheet and form three circles, making sure to press dough out evenly. Bake for 10 minutes, or until the edges are brown. Flip the crusts. Turn oven temperature to 375 degrees. On one half of each round, spread sauce and top with toppings, careful to stay at least an inch from the edges. Pile high with toppings (again, carefully staying away from edges). Around the edge of the crust, sprinkle a small amount of mozzarella cheese. Fold crust over and press edges together firmly with your fingers by pressing down to the pan, leaving slight indentations. (cheese will melt and help hold crust together as well). Bake for another 30 minutes, or until top is sufficiently golden-brown. Let rest for 5 minutes. Serve with marinara for dipping, or your favorite sauce.

Makes 3 calzones. Per shell (calculate for toppings): Calories: 131 Carbohydrates: 2 Fiber: 0 Protein: 38 Fat: 24

DESSERTS

I've got to write this down before I forget. I'm making my son's favorite cake for his birthday today. And I wanted to make a cake for me too! It's in the oven, so I don't know how it'll turn out yet...

First...my son's cake recipe:

Hedgehog's Yellow Cake
by Maryann Macdonald

3/4 cup sugar
1/2 cup butter
3 eggs
1 1/4 cup self-rising flour *
1 teaspoon vanilla extract (optional)

1. Ask an adult to set the oven to 350* F.
2. Butter a 9-inch round pan.
3. Mix butter and sugar together in a bowl.
4. Add eggs, one by one.
5. If desired, add vanilla.
6. Mix in flour.
7. Put batter into pan and bake for half an hour.
8. Eat warm with a glass of milk.

* I used all-purpose flour and added 1 1/2 teaspoons baking powder and 1/4 teaspoon of salt.

To make a glaze, I used 2 cups powdered sugar, then add a bit of water a little at a time until it's as thick as glaze, pour it onto the middle of the cake and spread it a bit. The rest will spread over the whole cake.

Then recipe adjusted to be low-carb and no sugar for Lisa:

Adjusted Hedgehog Cake

1/2 cup butter
14 packets of sugar-free sweetener, I used 6 Splenda and 8 Stevia
5 eggs
1/8 tsp cream of tar tar
1 tsp vanilla
1 1/4 cup almond meal
1 1/2 tsp baking powder
1/8 tsp salt

1. Set the oven to 300* F or 325* F.
2. Butter a 9-inch round pan.
3. Mix butter and sugar together in a bowl.
4. Separate eggs, yolks go in with the butter and sweetener.
5. To the whites, add cream of tartar and mix until white, no peaks, just white.
6. If desired, add vanilla.
7. Mix in almond meal, salt, and baking powder.
8. Add the egg white mixture.
9. Put batter into pan and bake for half an hour.

How did it come out? It was a bit dry, but I ate it anyway!

Avocado-Chocolate Pudding

I always want to eat dessert first ** who doesn't? Better yet is eating dessert for dinner.

Raw chocolate, often called cacao (ka-KOW), is the base ingredient for all chocolaty treats, but the cacao is usually cooked, processed and turned into the well-known cocoa, which is still tasty, but doesn't have the same amazing nutritional and energizing benefits.

One of my favorite healthy dessert recipes is avocado-chocolate pudding. It's literally so nutritious and filling that you can have it for dinner.

I never use measurements, so you'll have to figure everything to taste, but it*s really quite simple:

* 1 or 2 ripe, soft avocados (3/4 to 1 avocado per person)

* A few spoonfuls of raw cacao powder
* A few spoonfuls of natural sweetener (honey, agave nectar, or maple syrup)
*A dash of salt and a squeeze of lemon or lime juice
*A dash of cinnamon, to taste

Simple, fast, delicious! The avocado is a healthy and filling fat source, so you'll feel like you've had a real meal, and it*s such a diverse fruit, it can be eaten sweetened or salted. The cacao powder gives you energy and is high in anti-oxidants. The natural sweeteners make sure you get a slow, sustained rise in blood sugar (unlike refined white sugar, which causes a spike and a crash).

For my chocolate fix, I like Russell Stover's Dark Chocolate Sugar-Free chocolate bar. Here's a cute poem:

> Russell Stovers
> Candy's Dandy
> When no other
> Sweets are handy.
>
> Still, use caution
> Eating yours
> Or you're gonna
> Poop your drawers.

Yummy Strawberries & "Cream" ~Maintenance

1 Tbsp Cream Cheese
2 - 3 Tbsp milk
Stevia, to taste
5 - 6 strawberries, sliced
MIX MIX MIX until its like a "cream" ... then add strawberries and enjoy! Cathy says, The "cream" will still be kinda lumpy, but once you add the strawberries it will all mix together fine.

Cinnamon Mug Bread
1/4 C. Flaxseed Meal
1/2 Tsp. Baking Powder(i use a pinch of cream of tartar and a pinch of baking soda since baking powder has cornstarch in it which is not allowed in P3)
1 tsp. Cinnamon

1 Packet Stevia
1 Egg
1 teaspoon Butter or Coconut oil, softened

Mix dry ingredients in a small bowl. In a coffee mug mix wet ingredients and beat until smooth. Add dry ingredients and blend well. Cook in microwave or 1 1/2 - 2 minutes. Let it cool slightly and then slice up. Great with butter

Variation - add a few pieces of chopped apple

Chocolate bark
equal parts of coconut oil and unsweetened cocoa, if you want to make it coconut bark then just add unsweetened shredded coconut
a few drops of stevia
spread on parchment paper and refrigerate to cool

Chocolate Cheesecake Bites

1 cup heavy cream
2 tsp vanilla extract
1/2 tsp stevia extract (12 packets)
8 oz pkg Neufchatel cream cheese at room temperature
1/4 cup unsweetened cocoa powder

Freeze mixing bowl and beaters for 5 minutes. Sift cocoa powder. In deep bowl whip heavy cream until soft peaks for m. Add vanilla and 1/4 tsp stevia extract or 5 packets. In separate bowl mix cream cheese until soft using 2-3 tbsp whipping cream to thin cream cheese. Once cream cheese is smooth, add the cocoa powder and the other 1/4 tsp stevia extract. place mixer on high speed and add cream cheese mixture to whipped cream.

Put mini paper cups in small muffin tin and spray with canola oil. drop in cheesecake mixture by tablespoons. cover and place in freezer.

Oopsie Apple Pie

4 eggs, separated
4 oz cream cheese
1/8 tsp cream of tartar
1/4 tsp vanilla extract (make sure it has no sugar)
1 tsp stevia extract, divided
6 med size apples
2T unsalted butter
1 tsp cinnamon
pinch of salt (if using salted butter, omit)

Beat egg whites with cream of tartar until stiff peaks form. Mix egg yolk with cream cheese, vanilla, and 1/2 tsp stevia. Gently fold in yolk mixture to whites, half at a time. Divide mix into two greased round cake pans, (I used parchment paper, also greased, to aid in removal). Cook @ 300 for 30-35 min, until firmly set. Let cool for 5 min. Remove from pans and allow to cool completely.

Peel, core and slice apples. Melt butter in skillet and add cinnamon, 1/2 tsp stevia, and salt to melted butter. Add apples. Stir until well coated. Cover and cook until apples are tender. Be careful not to scorch them!

Peel parchment off oopsie rounds. Place one in bottom of glass pie plate. Spoon apple mix over top. Cover with remaining oopsie round, leaving the side that looks the best facing up. Slice as you would a normal pie, taking care, because it is delicate. Serve with sugar free whipped cream.

"Sex on P-Three"
(I use my Magic-Bullet mixer and cups to make these)

Ok you rum-lovers! ;) Recipe is as follows:

- 2-3 shots Parrot Bay coconut rum
(all rest are approx. or to taste:)
- 3/4c OJ
- 1/2 tbsp coconut extract
- 1/4c pineapple juice
- 1/2c fruit punch
- 1/2c crushed ice

Blend until smooth and enjoy!

Frozen "Maintenance-Rita" (strawberry)

-Crushed ice, fill halfway in a Magic Bullet mixer cup
-Three large frozen strawberries
-Two shots Jose Cuervo
-Two 1/2 shots lime juice
-One shot lemon juice
-One packet truvia or stevia (or to taste)

Blend and enjoy!
(Add 1 shot water if too strong)

Low-Carb, (gluten-free) Crullers (of the oopsie variety)

3 eggs, separated
3 ounces cream cheese
1 tsp baking powder
1/8 tsp cream of tartar
1 packet Splenda
2 Tbsp Davincis Vanilla Syrup (Sugar Free)

Preheat oven to 300 degrees F.

In a bowl, whip egg whites with cream of tartar until peaks are stiff (about 5 minutes).

In separate bowl, blend cream cheese, yolks, cream of tartar and davincis sugar free syrup. Adding half of the yolk batter at a time to the whites and using a tall spoon (I use an iced tea spoon), make a lazy sine wave through the batter once. Turn the bowl 90 degrees and repeat. Add second half of the yolk mix and repeat sine wave two more times.
Place in ungreased, nonstick angel food miniature cake pans.

Bake for 30 minutes. Remove pans from oven and let cool on a cooling rack. .Makes 4 crullers.

Chocolate Glaze

2 Lindt 80% dark chocolate squares (buy in candy bar)
1 Tbsp davincis vanilla sugar free syrup
2 small packets Splenda
2 Tbsp heavy whipping cream
2 Tbsp butter
In a microwavable bowl, combine ingredients. Microwave for 30 seconds. Stir well. Dip tops of crullers into mixture. Drizzle any remaining mixture to fill bare spots. Let crullers rest on cooling rack until glaze has set.

Will coat 6-8 crullers, and can be used for other purposes.
This does dry to a shiny glaze.

Keep unused portions and completes recipes in cooler temperatures.

Nutritional information for entire chocolate glaze recipe:

Calories: 349
Carbohydrates: 5
Fiber: 2
Net Carbohydrates: 3
Protein: 3
Fat: 36

Nutritional information without glaze/with glaze (glaze will easily coat 6-8 crullers):
Calories: 218/273
Carbohydrates: 2/1
Fiber: 0/1
Net Carbohydrates: 2/3
Protein: 7.5 grams/ 8 grams
Fat: 18 grams/ 24 grams

Angel Food Cake

3 eggs, separated
3 ounces cream cheese

1 tsp baking powder
1/8 tsp cream of tartar
1 packet Splenda
2 Tbsp Davincis Vanilla Syrup (Sugar Free)

1 cup whipping cream
3 packets Splenda
Frozen berries

Preheat oven to 300 degrees.

In a bowl, whip egg whites with cream of tartar until peaks are stiff (about 5 minutes).

In separate bowl, blend cream cheese, yolks, cream of tartar and davincis sugar free syrup. Adding half of the yolk batter at a time to the whites and using a tall spoon (I use an iced tea spoon), make a lazy sine wave through the batter once. Turn the bowl 90 degrees and repeat. Add second half of the yolk mix and repeat sine wave two more times.

In each non-greased pan, carefully spoon * of the batter, spreading about the edges. (If you only have 2 pans, you can refrigerate the batter for the next round.)

Bake for 30 minutes. Remove pans from oven and let cool on a cooling rack.

When ready to serve:
Arrange cooled cakes on plates.

In a bowl, whip heavy cream with two packets Splenda until still peaks form. Spoon cream into the center of each mini cake. Tuck fresh fruit in and on the cakes. Sprinkle one packet of Splenda along the top (optional).
Refrigerate leftovers.
Makes 4 mini cakes.
Nutritional information:
Calories: 218
Carbohydrates: 6
Fiber: 0
Net Carbohydrates: 6
Protein: 7.5 grams
Fat: 18 grams

Low Carb Crepes (of the Oopsie variety)

3 eggs, separated
3 ounces cream cheese
1 tsp baking powder
1/8 tsp cream of tartar
1 packet Splenda
2 Tbsp Davincis Vanilla Syrup (Sugar Free)
2 Tbsp canola oil

1 cup whipping cream
3 packets Splenda
Frozen berries

Preheat oil in skillet over medium-low heat.

In a bowl, whip egg whites with cream of tartar until peaks are stiff (about 5 minutes).

In separate bowl, blend cream cheese, yolks, cream of tartar and davincis sugar free syrup. Adding half of the yolk batter at a time to the whites and using a tall spoon (I use an iced tea spoon), make a lazy sine wave through the batter once. Turn the bowl 90 degrees and repeat. Add second half of the yolk mix and repeat sine wave two more times.

Using scant * cup scoop, drop batter onto heated pan. Let cook until bottom of the batter is firm about 3-5 minutes. Flip and press lightly. Let cook for another 1-2 minutes, until crepe is set. Move to a plate to cool.

When ready to serve:

Arrange crepes on a plate (best looking side down).

In a bowl, whip heavy cream with two packets Splenda until still peaks form. Spoon cream into the center of each crepe. Roll and place seam-side down. Tuck fresh fruit in, on and around the crepes. Sprinkle one packet of Splenda along the top (optional).

Refrigerate leftovers.

Makes 6 crepes.

Nutritional information:
Calories: 144
Carbohydrates: 4
Fiber: 0
Net Carbohydrates: 4
Protein: 5 grams
Fat: 12 grams

MORE LOW-CARB RECIPES

~not for the first 3 weeks of Maintenance…it's for the 2nd phase and beyond~

Raw Cheesecake

by Dr. Theresa Ramsey, The Center for Natural Healing

Crust Ingredients:
2 cups raw macadamia nuts
1/2 cup dates, pitted

Cheese Filling Ingredients:
3 cups chopped cashews (soaked for at least 1 hour, preferably overnight) ¾ cup lemon juice ½ to ¾ cup agave ¾ cup coconut oil (warmed to room temperature to clear liquid)
1 tsp. vanilla
½ - ¾ tsp. Celtic sea salt

Raspberry Dripping Sauce:
1 bag frozen raspberries
½ cup dates

Preparation of Crust: Process the macadamia nuts and dates in the food processor. Cut a piece of parchment paper for the bottom of a 9 inch spring form pan.
Roll out crust on top of the parchment paper.

Preparation of the Filling: Blend in a vitamixer the cashews that are starting to sprout, lemon, agave, coconut oil, vanilla, sea salt, and ½ cup water. Blend until smooth and adjust to taste.

Pour the mixture onto the crust. Remove air bubbles by tapping the pan on a table.
Place in the freezer until firm. Remove the whole cake from the pan while frozen and place on a serving platter. Defrost in the refrigerator.

Preparation of the Raspberry Sauce: Process raspberries and dates in a food processor until well blended.

Most of the fat and calories in this pie comes from coconut oil, cashews and macadamia nuts. There is just about an equal amount of saturated fats as there is unsaturated fat. These fats are fats that make you thin. It is known that a blend of fat intake (unsaturated and saturated) are satisfying to the taste buds as well as the belly fullness. They are slower to digest and therefore give more lasting satiation when ingested. The type of fat in coconuts, cashews and macadamia nuts are medium chain triglycerides which burn more efficiently than long chain triglycerides and therefore give the body more energy.

Totally Sinless Chocolate Cake

6 Tbsp. unsweetened cocoa powder
1 tsp. aluminum-free baking powder
½ tsp. baking soda
¾ c erythritol
6 Tbsp. unsalted organic butter or extra virgin coconut oil
5 large eggs
One 15 ounce can of black beans or 1 ½ c cooked beans (any color)

Spaghetti Squash Chicken Casserole

Makes 6 servings
Prep time: 15 minutes
Cook time: 1 hour unattended

5 cups cooked spaghetti squash
2 pounds of asparagus (use 4 cups of organic baby spinach in place of asparagus if you wish)
1 1/2 Tbsb olive oil
4-6 oz. organic chicken breasts, 6 oz, cut in half
2 tsp sea salt
2 28oz cans of low-sodium diced organic tomatoes*
2 Tbsp fresh thyme, chopped (1 Tbsp dried)
2 Tbsp fresh rosemary, chopped (1 Tbsp dried)
4 cloves garlic, chopped
Olive oil or olive oil cooking spray

1) Preheat oven to 350. Lightly brush or spray a 9 x 13" glass casserole dish with olive oil.
2) Spread squash into bottom of casserole dish
3) Place asparagus side by side across squash.
4) Drizzle 1 Tbsp olive oil over asparagus.
5) Rub or sprinkle 1/4 tsp salt onto each chicken breast half. Place chicken over asparagus.
6) Pour diced tomatoes over chicken.
7) Combine thyme, rosemary, and garlic and evenly sprinkle mixture over top.
8) Bake approximately 1 hour or until chicken center reaches 165 degrees.

* contact manufacturer to ensure product is gluten-free

45 calorie Chocolate Pudding

This pudding was so fast and easy to make. I can't believe it was only 45 calories!

To thicken the pudding, I used guar gum. Guar gum can best be described as a natural food thickener, similar to cornstarch. Guar gum has significantly more thickening ability than cornstarch, at a fraction of the cost; which is why you see this in the ingredients lists for many products such as puddings and ice creams. Until recently, guar gum was also an ingredient in non-prescription diet pills designed to create a sense of fullness. Guar gum thickens because the structure of it is an insoluble fiber.

Benefits of Guar Gum
* Lowering blood Glucose
* Lowering insulin levels

3/4 cup chocolate unsweetened almond milk
1/2 tsp guar gum or xanthan gum
1 TBS cocoa powder
Truvia to taste (or stevia glycerite)

Place in a medium sized bowl and blend until smooth. Let sit for 5 minutes to "set." The mixture will thicken up. Enjoy!

Nutritional Comparison:
JELL-O Fat-Free chocolate pudding = 93 calories, 21 carbs, 0.3 fiber
Almond milk pudding = 45 calories, 5 carbs, 2.7g fiber

3-Minute Chocolate Cake

Ingredients -
1/4C Almond flour
1 T Cocoa Power
1/4 t Baking Power
5 packets of Splenda (1 packet is about 2 teaspoons of sugar, so use whatever sweetener you like)

2 T Melted Butter
1 T Water
1 Egg

In a microwave-safe bowl, blend all dry ingredients. Add water, melted butter and egg...mix throughly. Cover with plastic wrap, cutting a small slit in center of plastic wrap to vent. Microwave on high for 1 minute or a little longer. Let it cool a bit.

Instead of Splenda packets which contain maltodextrin, you can use SF flavored syrups like DaVinci. Just omit the water if you use a syrup. Of course you can use Stevia or Erythritol.

Gluten Free Pumpkin Muffins

Gluten Free Coconut Flour Pumpkin Muffins recipe photo
Gluten Free Coconut Flour Pumpkin Muffins
Prepared by Sarah Shilhavy, Photo by Jeremiah Shilhavy

Servings: 12 muffins
Preparation time: 10 minutes

* 1/2 cup coconut flour
* 1/2 teaspoon baking powder
* 1 teaspoon cinnamon powder
* 1/4 teaspoon cloves
* 1/4 teaspoon allspice/nutmeg
* 1/2 cup pumpkin puree
* 6 eggs (or 4 whole eggs and 2 whites...a good way to use up your egg whites)
* 1 teaspoon vanilla
* 1/2 cup coconut oil, melted
* 3/8 cup maple syrup (about 3 1/2 oz)
* pinch salt
* 1/4 cup chopped walnut pieces

Preheat oven to 400F. Grease a muffin pan or line with paper liners.

Sift together coconut flour and spices together.

Whisk remaining ingredients together (except walnuts) in a separate bowl until well mixed.

With a wooden spoon or whisk stir the flour mixture gradually into the pumpkin mixture so that no lumps remain.

Divide batter between 12 muffin cups. Sprinkle with walnuts.

Bake for 12 minutes or until toothpick inserted in center comes out clean. Do not over bake as the flour can burn easily. Frost with icing once cool (optional).

<u>Cream Cheese Icing</u>

* 8 oz cream cheese, softened
* 1/2 cup butter, softened
* 1/4 cup maple syrup or honey
* 1 teaspoon vanilla extract

Combine all ingredients together into a small bowl. Beat with an electric mixer until well mixed and light and fluffy.

Flour-less Chocolate Tiramisu Torte

Chocolate Torte:
7 ounces unsweetened chocolate
1 ¾ sticks salted butter
...1 ¼ cup TRUVIA or erythritol
2 TBS Stevia Glycerite (omit if using Truvia)
5 large eggs

Mascarpone filling:
1 8-ounce package mascarpone (or cream cheese)
4 TBS Truvia (or 1 tsp stevia glycerite)...to taste
1 egg

Preheat oven to 375 degrees. Grease a muffin tin pan. Set aside.Brown the butter (if desired...tastes way better!) in a saucepan. Once the butter is brown (not black!), slowly add the chocolate. Add the sweetener. Let cool in fridge for awhile. Once cool, add one egg at a time. Cream filling: Mix mascarpone cheese, sweetener and egg. Fill the muffin tins with chocolate filling and a dollop of cheese in the middle. Bake for 25 minutes. Enjoy!

Makes 16 servings
Nutritional Info (per serving) = 212 calories, 4.1 carbs, 2 fiber

Artichoke "Rice" Salad

1/2 cup chicken stock
6 cups "riced" cauliflower
1 tsp curry powder
...(tharr be more)salt and pepper to taste
5 green onions, chopped
1 green bell pepper, chopped
3 stalks celery, chopped
3 (6.5 ounce) jars marinated artichoke hearts, chopped
1 cup homemade olive oil mayonnaise
1/4 cup chopped parsley

Combine chicken stock and cauliflower rice in a medium saucepan. Cook until tender, about 3 minutes. Then drain any excess liquid. In a small bowl, mix together artichoke marinade, mayonnaise, and curry powder. Season to taste with salt and pepper. Set aside. In a large bowl, combine artichoke hearts, green onions, green bell pepper, parsley, and celery. Mix in "rice", then mix in reserved marinade mixture. Cover and chill overnight. Serve cold. Makes 12 servings.

NUTRITIONAL COMPARISON (per serving):
Traditional Artichoke Rice Salad = 468 calories, 31.6 carbs, 1.1g fiber (30.5 effective carbs)
"Healthified" Rice Salad = 192 calories, 10.8 carbs, 8.1g fiber (2.7 effective carbs)

Peanut Butter Twix

Ingredients in a Traditional TWIX bar = Milk Chocolate (Sugar, Cocoa Butter, Milk Ingredients, Cocoa Mass, Lactose, Soy Lecithin, Polyglycerol Polyricinoleate, Artificial Flavour)Enriched Flour (Flour, Niacin, Reduced Iron, Thiamine Mononitrate, Riboflavin, Folic Acid)Sugar, Hydrolyzed Palm and Palm Kernel Oil, Corn ...Syrup, Milk Ingredients, Dextrose, Salt, Cocoa Mass, Sodium Bicarbonate, Soy Lecithin, Soybean Oil, Artificial Flavor.

Try this instead...
Cookie Layer:

1/2 cup vanilla whey (Jay Robb...no sugar)
3/4 cup almond flour
1/4 tsp baking soda
1/4 tsp Celtic sea salt
1/4 cup butter or coconut oil
4 TBS Truvia (or erythritol and a few drops stevia glycerite)
1-2 TBS vanilla almond milk OR water (just enough to hold dough together)

Preheat the oven to 375 degrees F. In a medium bowl, stir together the whey, almond flour, baking soda and salt. Cut in the butter using a pastry blender or your fingers until the butter lumps are smaller than peas. Stir in the almond milk and sweetener to form a stiff dough. Take about 2 TBS of dough at a time to roll out long biscuit shapes (resembling a Twix bar). Place on cookie sheet. Bake for 7 minutes, turn off oven. Leave in oven for 3 more minutes to cool to crisp up. Place in freezer to freeze (frozen biscuits will hold the caramel better).

Peanut Butter Layer:
6 TBS Natural Peanut Butter
6 TBS vanilla almond milk
Sweetener to taste

Place all ingredients in a mixing bowl and stir until well combined. Add sweetener to taste. Place peanut butter sauce on top of the cookie and place in freezer to set.

Chocolate:
1 CHOCO-Perfection OR Simply Lite Bar
2 TBS vanilla almond milk

In a microwavable bowl, combine ingredients. Microwave for 30 seconds. Stir well. Drizzle over the peanut butter covered cookie. Place in freezer to set. Makes 12 individual twix bars.

NUTRITIONAL COMPARISON (per 2 Twix bars)
Traditional Twix = 290 calories, 37 carbs, 1g fiber
"Healthified" Twix = 235 calories, 5 carbs, 3.25g fiber

Guacamole "Angel" Eggs

Instead of mayo in your Deviled Eggs, try avocado! YUM!!!

10 hardboiled eggs, peeled and sliced length-wise
1 teaspoon Dijon mustard
1 teaspoon minced hot pepper
1 teaspoon minced onion
1 small avocado
baby cherry tomato halves (for garnish)

In a bowl mix together all ingredients. Spoon an equal amount into each of the egg halves. Top each with a baby tomato half. Enjoy

Chocolate PB Stuffed Teddy Grahams

1/2 cup vanilla whey (Jay Robb...no sugar)
3/4 cup almond flour*
1/4 tsp baking soda
...1/4 tsp Celtic sea salt
1/4 cup unsweetened cocoa powder
1/4 cup NATURAL almond or peanut butter
4 TBS Truvia (or erythritol and a drop of stevia glycerite)
2 TBS water (just enough to hold dough together)

Preheat the oven to 400 degrees F (200 degrees C). In a medium bowl, stir together the whey, almond flour (*doesn't need to be blanched), cocoa powder, baking soda and salt. Cut in the peanut butter using a pastry blender or your fingers until the butter lumps are smaller than peas. Stir in the water and sweetener to form a stiff dough. On parchment paper (lightly greased), roll the dough out to 1/8 inch in thickness. Cut into desired shapes with cookie cutters. Place cookies 1 inch apart onto cookie sheets. Bake for 5 to 7 minutes in the preheated oven, until edges are lightly browned. Remove from cookie sheets to cool on wire racks.

Filling:
1/2 cup natural almond or peanut butter
1/2 cup cream cheese
Stevia Glycerite (to taste) or 2 packets of Truvia

Mix together and use to hold cookies together:) Makes 24 mini sandwich cookies.

Nutritional Information (per 2 sandwich cookies) = 178 calories, 3.8 carbs, 1.4g fiber

Pecan Coconut Macaroons with Chocolate Ganache

3 large egg whites
1/4 tsp salt
1/4 vanilla extract
1/8 tsp cream of tartar
3/4 cup granulated erythritol (or granulated sugar)
1 tbsp agave nectar
1 1/4 cup unsweetened, shredded coconut
1/2 cup finely ground pecans
3 tbsp butter
1 85% cacao Lindt bar, chopped (or 3.5 oz chocolate of your choice)

Preheat the oven to 325F and line two baking sheets with parchment paper.

In a large bowl, whip egg whites with salt, vanilla and cream of tarter until they are frothy. With the beater running, slowly add erythritol or sugar and agave nectar and keep beating until stiff peaks form. Gently fold in coconut and ground pecans.

Drop by small spoonfuls onto prepared baking sheets. Use the spoon to create a well in the center of each macaroon and build up the sides. Bake for 20 minutes, or until golden brown. Turn off oven and prop open the door with a wooden spoon and let the macaroons cool in oven for about an hour.

In a small metal or ceramic bowl set over a pot of gently simmering water, melt butter and chocolate together. Stir until smooth. Drop spoonfuls of melted chocolate into the center of each macaroon. Let cool until set.

Makes 24 cookies. Each cookie has a total of 9.2g of carbs, but only 3.2 if you subtract erythritol.

Easy Almond Joys

2 TBS coconut oil (melted)
2 TBS unsweetened cocoa powder
1 TBS almond butter
1 TBS coconut flour
Stevia glycerite (optional to taste...I didn't use any)

Mix cocoa into the coconut oil. Then add in the almond butter, mix until smooth. Then add the coconut flour (and sweetener if desired). Pour into mini ice cube trays. Freeze for at least 5-6 minutes and either store in the fridge or freezer. Makes 4 servings.

NUTRITIONAL COMPARISON (per serving)
Traditional Almond Joys = 235 calories, 29.2 carbs, 2.5g fiber
"Healthified" Almond Joys = 88.5 calories, 3.6 carbs, 1.7 fiber

Coconut Banana Cookies

 I made these for the first time today and the one thing I learned from the first batch is that the cookies don't spread out like traditional dough so you have to shape them how you want them to cook. With my first batch I made little balls so I ended up with ball cookies so for the second batch I shaped them into little balls and then smashed them a bit to shape them into an actual cookie.

INGREDIENTS:
1/2 cup + 1 tablespoon coconut flour
1/2 teaspoon baking soda

8 tablespoons refined coconut oil (I melted for 30 seconds in the microwave before adding to the bowl)

2 large eggs
1 very ripe banana
1 1/2 teaspoons vanilla
3/4 cup dark chocolate chips

INSTRUCTIONS
-In a medium bowl whisk the coconut flour and the baking soda together.
- In a large bowl mix together the coconut oil, banana, eggs, and vanilla.
- Then mix the dry ingredients into the wet.
- Add the chocolate chips.

- Bake at 350 for 12 minutes.
- Enjoy!

Cream of "WHEAT"

¾ cup of warm unsweetened vanilla or chocolate almond milk
2 TBS freshly ground golden flaxseeds (or more for a thicker "cereal")
1 tsp psyllium husk
1 scoop vanilla or chocolate egg white/whey protein
1 TBS vanilla extract
1 drop of stevia glycerite
½ tsp of nutmeg
½ tsp cinnamon
Optional: you can add some coconut flakes, nuts or peanut butter to this recipe.

Combine warm milk, flax, whey, stevia, cinnamon and nutmeg (and other toppings) in a bowl. Stir well and let sit for a few minutes until the "oatmeal" thickens. Enjoy!

NUTRITIONAL COMPARISON (per serving):
Traditional Cream of Wheat with Skim Milk = 230 calories, 39.6 carbs, 1.3 fiber, 12 protein
"Healthified" Cream of Wheat = 230 calories, 5g carbs, 4g fiber, 29g protein

Micah's favorite treat

1 can coconut milk
1 cup smooth almond butter
1/2 cup Jay Robb vanilla whey protein

In a blender, mix until smooth (you can add more whey or coconut flour to thicken it more). I store in the fridge for an easy dessert.
*from Maria Mind Body Health

The following is the Dr. Simeon's manuscript written in 1954:

Pounds & Inches

A NEW APPROACH TO OBESITY

BY: DR. A.T.W. SIMEONS

SALVATOR MUNDI INTERNATIONAL HOSPITAL
00152 - ROME VIALE MURA GIANICOLENSI, 77.

FOREWORD

This book discusses a new interpretation of the nature of obesity, and while it does not advocate yet another fancy slimming diet it does describe a method of treatment which has grown out of theoretical considerations based on clinical observation.

What I have to say is an essence of views distilled out of forty years of grappling with the fundamental problems of obesity, its causes, its symptoms, and its very nature. In these many years of specialized work thousands of cases have passed through my hands and were carefully studied. Every new theory, every new method, every promising lead was considered, experimentally screened and critically evaluated as soon as it became known. But invariably the results were disappointing and lacking in uniformity.

I felt that we were merely nibbling at the fringe of a great problem, as, indeed, do most serious students of overweight. We have grown pretty sure that the tendency to accumulate abnormal fat is a very definite metabolic disorder, much as is, for instance, diabetes. Yet the localization and the nature of this disorder remained a mystery. Every new approach seemed to lead into a blind alley, and though patients were told that they are fat because they eat too much, we believed that this is neither the whole truth nor the last word in the matter.

Refusing to be side-tracked by an all too facile interpretation of obesity, I have always held that overeating is the result of the disorder, not its cause, and that we can make little headway until we can build for ourselves some sort of theoretical structure with which to explain the condition. Whether such a structure represents the truth is not important at this moment. What it must do is to give us an intellectually satisfying interpretation of what is happening in the obese body. It must also be able to withstand the onslaught of all hitherto known clinical facts and furnish a hard background against which the results of treatment can be accurately assessed.

To me this requirement seems basic, and it has always been the center of my interest. In dealing with obese patients it became a habit to register and order every clinical experience as if it were an odd looking piece of a jig-saw puzzle. And then, as in a jig saw puzzle, little clusters of fragments began to form, though they seemed to fit in nowhere. As the years passed these clusters grew bigger and started to amalgamate until, about sixteen years ago, a complete picture became dimly discernible. This picture was, and still is, dotted with gaps for which I cannot find the pieces, but I do now feel that a theoretical structure is visible as a whole.

With mounting experience, more and more facts seemed to fit snugly into the new framework, and when then a treatment based on such speculations showed consistently satisfactory results, I was sure that some practical advance had been made, regardless of whether the theoretical interpretation of these results is correct or not.

The clinical results of the new treatment have been published in scientific journal and these reports have been generally well received by the profession, but the very nature of a scientific article does not permit the full presentation of new theoretical concepts nor is there room to discuss the finer points of technique and the reasons for observing them.

During the 16 years that have elapsed since I first published my findings, I have had many hundreds of inquiries from research institutes, doctors and patients. Hitherto I could only refer those interested to my scientific papers, though I realized that these did not contain sufficient information to enable doctors to conduct the new treatment satisfactorily. Those who tried were obliged to gain their own experience through the many trials and errors which I have long since overcome.

Doctors from all over the world have come to Italy to study the method, first hand in my clinic in the Salvator Mundi International Hospital in Rome. For some of them the time they could spare has been too short to get a full grasp of the technique, and in any case the number of those whom I have been able to meet personally is small compared with the many requests for further detailed information which keep coming in. I have tried to keep up with these demands by correspondence, but the volume of this work has become unmanageable and that is one excuse for writing this book.

In dealing with a disorder in which the patient must take an active part in the treatment, it is, I believe, essential that he or she have an understanding of what is being done and why. Only then can there be intelligent cooperation between physician and patient. In order to avoid writing two books, one for the physician and another for the patient - a prospect which would probably have resulted in no book at all - I have tried to meet the requirements of both in a single book. This is a rather difficult enterprise in which I may not have succeeded. The expert will grumble about long-windedness while the lay-reader may occasionally have to look up an unfamiliar word in the glossary provided for him. To make the text more readable I shall be unashamedly authoritative and avoid all the hedging and tentativeness with which it is customary to express new scientific concepts grown out of clinical experience and not as yet confirmed by clear-cut laboratory experiments. Thus, when I make what reads like a factual statement, the professional reader may have to translate into: clinical experience seems to suggest that such and such an observation might be tentatively explained by such and such a working hypothesis, requiring a vast amount of further research before the hypothesis can be considered a valid theory. If we can from the outset establish this as a mutually accepted convention, I hope to avoid being accused of speculative exuberance.

THE NATURE OF OBESITY

Obesity a Disorder

As a basis for our discussion we postulate that obesity in all its many forms is due to an abnormal functioning of some part of the body and that every ounce of abnormally accumulated fat is always the result of the same disorder of certain regulatory mechanisms. Persons suffering from this particular disorder will get fat regardless of whether they eat excessively, normally or less than normal. A person who is free of the disorder will never get fat, even if he frequently overeats.

Those in whom the disorder is severe will accumulate fat very rapidly, those in whom it is moderate will gradually increase in weight and those in whom it is mild may be able to keep their excess weight stationary for long periods. In all these cases a loss of weight brought about by dieting, treatments with thyroid, appetite-reducing drugs, laxatives, violent exercise, massage, baths, etc., is only temporary and will be rapidly regained as soon as the reducing regimen is relaxed. The reason is simply that none of these measures corrects the basic disorder.

While there are great variations in the severity of obesity, we shall consider all the different forms in both sexes and at all ages as always being due to the same disorder. Variations in form would then be partly a matter of degree, partly an inherited bodily constitution and partly the result of a secondary involvement of endocrine glands such as the pituitary, the thyroid, the adrenals or the sex glands. On the other hand, we postulate that no deficiency of any of these glands can ever directly produce the common disorder known as obesity.

If this reasoning is correct, it follows that a treatment aimed at curing the disorder must be equally effective in both sexes, at all ages and in all forms of obesity. Unless this is so, we are entitled to harbor grave doubts as to whether a given treatment corrects the underlying disorder. Moreover, any claim that the disorder has been corrected must be substantiated by the ability of the patient to eat normally of any food he pleases without regaining abnormal fat after treatment. Only if these conditions are fulfilled can we legitimately speak of curing obesity rather than of reducing weight.

Our problem thus presents itself as an enquiry into the localization and the nature of the disorder which leads to obesity. The history of this enquiry is a long series of high hopes and bitter disappointments.

The History of Obesity

There was a time, not so long ago, when obesity was considered a sign of health and prosperity in man and of beauty, amorousness and fecundity in women. This attitude probably dates back to Neolithic times, about 8000 years ago; when for the first time in the history of culture, man began to own property, domestic animals, arable land, houses, pottery and metal tools. Before that, with the possible exception of some races such as the Hottentots, obesity was almost non-existent, as it still is in all wild animals and most primitive races.

Today obesity is extremely common among all civilized races, because a disposition to the disorder can be inherited. Wherever abnormal fat was regarded as an asset, sexual selection tended to propagate the trait. It is only in very recent times that manifest obesity has lost some of its allure, though the cult of the outsize bust - always a sign of latent obesity - shows that the trend still lingers on.

The Significance of Regular Meals

In the early Neolithic times another change took place which may well account for the fact that today nearly all inherited dispositions sooner or later develop into manifest obesity. This change was the institution of regular meals. In pre-Neolithic times, man ate only when he was hungry and only as much as he required to still the pangs of hunger. Moreover, much of his food was raw and all of it was unrefined. He roasted his meat, but he did not boil it, as he had no pots, and what little he may have grubbed from the Earth and picked from the trees, he ate as he went along.

The whole structure of man's omnivorous digestive tract is, like that of an ape, rat or pig, adjusted to the continual nibbling of tidbits. It is not suited to occasional gorging as is, for instance, the intestine of the carnivorous cat family. Thus the institution of regular meals, particularly of food rendered rapidly assimilable, placed a great burden on modern man's ability to cope with large quantities of food suddenly pouring into his system from the intestinal tract.

The institution of regular meals meant that man had to eat more than his body required at the moment of eating so as to tide him over until the next meal. Food rendered easily digestible suddenly flooded his body with nourishment of which he was in no need at the moment. Somehow, somewhere this surplus had to be stored.

Three Kinds of Fat

In the human body we can distinguish three kinds of fat. The first is the structural fat which fills the gaps between various organs, a sort of packing material. Structural fat also performs such important functions as bedding the kidneys in soft elastic tissue, protecting the coronary arteries and keeping the skin smooth and taut. It also provides the springy cushion of hard fat under the bones of the feet, without which we would be unable to walk.

The second type of fat is a normal reserve of fuel upon which the body can freely draw when the nutritional income from the intestinal tract is insufficient to meet the demand. Such normal reserves are localized all over the body. Fat is a substance which packs the highest caloric value into the smallest space so that normal reserves of fuel for muscular activity and the maintenance of body temperature can be most economically stored in this form. Both these types of fat, structural and reserve, are normal, and even if the body stocks them to capacity this can never be called obesity.

But there is a third type of fat which is entirely abnormal. It is the accumulation of such fat, and of such fat only, from which the overweight patient suffers. This abnormal fat is also a potential reserve of fuel, but unlike the normal reserves it is not available to the body in a nutritional emergency. It is, so to speak, locked away in a fixed deposit and is not kept in a current account, as are the normal reserves.

When an obese patient tries to reduce by starving himself, he will first lose his normal fat reserves. When these are exhausted he begins to burn up structural fat, and only as a last resort will the body yield its abnormal reserves, though by that time the patient usually feels so weak and hungry that the diet is abandoned. It is just for this reason that obese patients complain that when they diet they lose the wrong fat. They feel famished and tired and their face becomes drawn and haggard, but their belly, hips, thighs and upper arms show little improvement. The fat they have come to detest stays on and the fat they need to cover their bones gets less and less. Their skin wrinkles and they look old and miserable. And that is one of the most frustrating and depressing experiences a human being can have.

Injustice to the Obese

When then obese patients are accused of cheating, gluttony, lack of will power, greed and sexual complexes, the strong become indignant and decide that modern medicine is a fraud and its representatives fools, while the weak just give up the struggle in despair. In either case the result is the same: a further gain in weight, resignation to an abominable fate and the resolution at least to live tolerably the short span allotted to them - a fig for doctors and insurance companies.

Obese patients only feel physically well as long as they are stationary or gaining weight. They may feel guilty, owing to the lethargy and indolence always associated with obesity. They may feel ashamed of what they have been led to believe is a lack of control. They may feel horrified by the appearance of their nude body and the tightness of their clothes. But they have a primitive feeling of animal content which turns to misery and suffering as soon as they make a resolute attempt to reduce. For this there are sound reasons.

In the first place, more caloric energy is required to keep a large body at a certain temperature than to heat a small body. Secondly the muscular effort of moving a heavy body is greater than in the case of a light body. The muscular effort consumes Calories which must be provided by food. Thus, all other factors being equal, a fat person requires more food than a lean one. One might therefore reason that if a fat person eats only the additional food his body requires he should be able to keep his weight stationary. Yet every physician who has studied obese patients under rigorously controlled conditions knows that this is not true.

Many obese patients actually gain weight on a diet which is calorically deficient for their basic needs. There must thus be some other mechanism at work.

Glandular Theories
At one time it was thought that this mechanism might be concerned with the sex glands. Such a connection was suggested by the fact that many juvenile obese patients show an under-development of the sex organs. The middle-age spread in men and the tendency of many women to put on weight in the menopause seemed to indicate a causal connection between diminishing sex function and overweight. Yet, when highly active sex hormones became available, it was found that their administration had no effect whatsoever on obesity. The sex glands could therefore not be the seat of the disorder.

The Thyroid Gland
When it was discovered that the thyroid gland controls the rate at which body-fuel is consumed, it was thought that by administering thyroid gland to obese patients their abnormal fat deposits could be burned up more rapidly. This too proved to be entirely disappointing, because as we now know, these abnormal deposits take no part in the body's energy-turnover - they are inaccessibly locked away. Thyroid medication merely forces the body to consume its normal fat reserves, which are already depleted in obese patients, and then to break down structurally essential fat without touching the abnormal deposits. In this way a patient may be brought to the brink of starvation in spite of having a hundred pounds of fat to spare. Thus any weight loss brought about by thyroid medication is always at the expense of fat of which the body is in dire need.

While the majority of obese patients have a perfectly normal thyroid gland and some even have an overactive thyroid, one also occasionally sees a case with a real thyroid deficiency. In such cases, treatment with thyroid brings about a small loss of weight, but this is not due to the loss of any abnormal fat. It is entirely the result of the elimination of a mucoid substance, called myxedema, which the body accumulates when there is a marked primary thyroid deficiency. Moreover, patients suffering only from a severe lack of thyroid hormone never become obese in the true sense. Possibly also the observation that normal persons - though not the obese - lose weight rapidly when their thyroid becomes overactive may have contributed to the false notion that thyroid deficiency and obesity are connected. Much misunderstanding about the supposed role of the thyroid gland in obesity is still met with, and it is now really high time that thyroid preparations be once and for all struck off the list of remedies for obesity. This is particularly so because giving thyroid gland to an obese patient whose thyroid is either normal or overactive, besides being useless, is decidedly dangerous.

The Pituitary Gland

The next gland to be falsely incriminated was the anterior lobe of the pituitary, or hypophysis. This most important gland lies well protected in a bony capsule at the base of the skull. It has a vast number of functions in the body, among which is the regulation of all the other important endocrine glands. The fact that various signs of anterior pituitary deficiency are often associated with obesity raised the hope that the seat of the disorder might be in this gland. But although a large number of pituitary hormones have been isolated and many extracts of the gland prepared, not a single one or any combination of such factors proved to be of any value in the treatment of obesity. Quite recently, however, a fat-mobilizing factor has been found in pituitary glands, but it is still too early to say whether this factor is destined to play a role in the treatment of obesity.

The Adrenals

Recently, a long series of brilliant discoveries concerning the working of the adrenal or suprarenal glands, small bodies which sit atop the kidneys, have created tremendous interest. This interest also turned to the problem of obesity when it was discovered that a condition which in some respects resembles a severe case of obesity - the so called Cushing's Syndrome - was caused by a glandular new-growth of the adrenals or by their excessive stimulation with ACTH, which is the pituitary hormone governing the activity of the outer rind or cortex of the adrenals.

When we learned that an abnormal stimulation of the adrenal cortex could produce signs that resemble true obesity, this knowledge furnished no practical means of treating obesity by decreasing the activity of the adrenal cortex. There is no evidence to suggest that in obesity there is any excess of adrenocortical activity; in fact, all the evidence points to the contrary. There seems to be rather a lack of adrenocortical function and a decrease in the secretion of ACTH from the anterior pituitary lobe.

So here again our search for the mechanism which produces obesity led us into a blind alley. Recently, many students of obesity have reverted to the nihilistic attitude that obesity is caused simply by overeating and that it can only be cured by under eating.

The Diencephalon or Hypothalamus

For those of us who refused to be discouraged there remained one slight hope. Buried deep down in the massive human brain there is a part which we have in common with all vertebrate animals the so-called diencephalon. It is a very primitive part of the brain and has in man been almost smothered by the huge masses of nervous tissue with which we think, reason and voluntarily move our body. The diencephalon is the part from which the central nervous system controls all the automatic animal functions of the body, such as breathing, the heart beat, digestion, sleep, sex, the urinary system, the autonomous or vegetative nervous system and via the pituitary the whole interplay of the endocrine glands.

It was therefore not unreasonable to suppose that the complex operation of storing and issuing fuel to the body might also be controlled by the diencephalon. It has long been known that the content of sugar - another form of fuel - in the blood depends on a certain nervous center in the diencephalon. When this center is destroyed in laboratory animals, they develop a condition rather similar to human stable diabetes. It has also long been known that the destruction of another diencephalic center produces a voracious appetite and a rapid gain in weight in animals which never get fat spontaneously.

The Fat-bank

Assuming that in man such a center controlling the movement of fat does exist, its function would have to be much like that of a bank. When the body assimilates from the intestinal tract more fuel than it needs at the moment, this surplus is deposited in what may be compared with a current account. Out of this account it can always be withdrawn as required. All normal fat reserves are in such a current account, and it is probable that a diencephalic center manages the deposits and withdrawals.

When now, for reasons which will be discussed later, the deposits grow rapidly while small withdrawals become more frequent, a point may be reached which goes beyond the diencephalon's banking capacity. Just as a banker might suggest to a wealthy client that instead of accumulating a large and unmanageable current account he should invest his surplus capital, the body appears to establish a fixed deposit into which all surplus funds go but from which they can no longer be withdrawn by the procedure used in a current account. In this way the diencephalic "fat-bank" frees itself from all work which goes beyond its normal banking capacity. The onset of obesity dates from the moment the diencephalon adopts this labor-saving ruse. Once a fixed deposit has been established the normal fat reserves are held at a minimum, while every available surplus is locked away in the fixed deposit and is therefore taken out of normal circulation.

THREE BASIC CAUSES OF OBESITY:

The Inherited Factor

Assuming that there is a limit to the diencephalon's fat banking capacity, it follows that there are three basic ways in which obesity can become manifest. The first is that the fat-banking capacity is abnormally low from birth. Such a congenitally low diencephalic capacity would then represent the inherited factor in obesity. When this abnormal trait is markedly present, obesity will develop at an early age in spite of normal feeding; this could explain why among brothers and sisters eating the same food at the same table some become obese and others do not.

Other Diencephalic Disorders

The second way in which obesity can become established is the lowering of a previously normal fat-banking capacity owing to some other diencephalic disorder. It seems to be a general rule that when one of the many diencephalic centers is particularly overtaxed; it tries to increase its capacity at the expense of other centers.

In the menopause and after castration the hormones previously produced in the sex-glands no longer circulate in the body. In the presence of normally functioning sex-glands their hormones act as a brake on the secretion of the sex-gland stimulating hormones of the anterior pituitary. When this brake is removed the anterior pituitary enormously increases its output of these sex-gland stimulating hormones, though they are now no longer effective. In the absence of any response from the non-functioning or missing sex glands, there is nothing to stop the anterior pituitary from producing more and more of these hormones. This situation causes an excessive strain on the diencephalic center which controls the function of the anterior pituitary. In order to cope with this additional burden the center appears to draw more and more energy away from other centers, such as those concerned with emotional stability, the blood circulation (hot flushes) and other autonomous nervous regulations, particularly also from the not so vitally important fat-bank.

The so-called stable type of diabetes heavily involves the diencephalic blood sugar regulating center. The diencephalon tries to meet this abnormal load by switching energy destined for the fat bank over to the sugar-regulating center, with the result that the fat-banking capacity is reduced to the point at which it is forced to establish a fixed deposit and thus initiate the disorder we call obesity. In this case one would have to consider the diabetes the primary cause of the obesity, but it is also possible that the process is reversed in the sense that a deficient or overworked fat-center draws energy from the sugar-center, in which case the obesity would be the cause of that type of diabetes in which the pancreas is not primarily involved. Finally, it is conceivable that in Cushing's syndrome those symptoms which resemble obesity are entirely due to the withdrawal of energy from the diencephalic fat-bank in order to make it available to the highly disturbed center which governs the anterior pituitary adrenocortical system.

Whether obesity is caused by a marked inherited deficiency of the fat-center or by some entirely different diencephalic regulatory disorder, its insurgence obviously has nothing to do with overeating and in either case obesity is certain to develop regardless of dietary restrictions. In these cases any enforced food deficit is made up from essential fat reserves and normal structural fat, much to the disadvantage of the patient's general health.

3)   The Exhaustion of the Fat-bank

But there is still a third way in which obesity can become established, and that is when a presumably normal fat-center is suddenly -- the emphasis is on suddenly -- called upon to deal with an enormous influx of food far in excess of momentary requirements. At first glance it does seem that here we have a straight-forward case of overeating being responsible for obesity, but on further analysis it soon becomes clear that the relation of cause and effect is not so simple. In the first place we are merely assuming that the capacity of the fat center is normal while it is possible and even probable that only persons who have some inherited trait in this direction can become obese merely by overeating.

Secondly, in many of these cases the amount of food eaten remains the same and it is only the consumption of fuel which is suddenly decreased, as when an athlete is confined to bed for many weeks with a broken bone or when a man leading a highly active life is suddenly tied to his desk in an office and to television at home. Similarly, when a person, grown up in a cold climate, is transferred to a tropical country and continues to eat as before, he may develop obesity because in the heat far less fuel is required to maintain the normal body temperature.

When a person suffers a long period of privation, be it due to chronic illness, poverty, famine or the exigencies of war, his diencephalic regulations adjust themselves to some extent to the low food intake. When then suddenly these conditions change and he is free to eat all the food he wants, this is liable to overwhelm his fat-regulating center. During the last war about 6000 grossly underfed Polish refugees who had spent harrowing years in Russia were transferred to a camp in India where they were well housed, given normal British army rations and some cash to buy a few extras. Within about three months, 85% were suffering from obesity.

In a person eating coarse and unrefined food, the digestion is slow and only a little nourishment at a time is assimilated from the intestinal tract. When such a person is suddenly able to obtain highly refined foods such as sugar, white flour, butter and oil these are so rapidly digested and assimilated that the rush of incoming fuel which occurs at every meal may eventually overpower the diecenphalic regulatory mechanisms and thus lead to obesity. This is commonly seen in the poor man who suddenly becomes rich enough to buy the more expensive refined foods, though his total caloric intake remains the same or is even less than before.

Psychological Aspects

Much has been written about the psychological aspects of obesity. Among its many functions the diencephalon is also the seat of our primitive animal instincts, and just as in an emergency it can switch energy from one center to another, so it seems to be able to transfer pressure from one instinct to another. Thus, a lonely and unhappy person deprived of all emotional comfort and of all instinct gratification except the stilling of hunger and thirst can use these as outlets for pent up instinct pressure and so develop obesity. Yet once that has happened, no amount of psychotherapy or analysis, happiness, company or the gratification of other instincts will correct the condition.

Compulsive Eating

No end of injustice is done to obese patients by accusing them of compulsive eating, which is a form of diverted sex gratification. Most obese patients do not suffer from compulsive eating; they suffer genuine hunger - real, gnawing, torturing hunger - which has nothing whatever to do with compulsive eating. Even their sudden desire for sweets is merely the result of the experience that sweets, pastries and alcohol will most rapidly of all foods allay the pangs of hunger. This has nothing to do with diverted instincts.

On the other hand, compulsive eating does occur in some obese patients, particularly in girls in their late teens or early twenties. Compulsive eating differs fundamentally from the obese patient's greater need for food. It comes on in attacks and is never associated with real hunger, a fact which is readily admitted by the patients. They only feel a feral desire to stuff. Two pounds of chocolates may be devoured in a few minutes; cold, greasy food from the refrigerator, stale bread, leftovers on stacked plates, almost anything edible is crammed down with terrifying speed and ferocity.

I have occasionally been able to watch such an attack without the patient's knowledge, and it is a frightening, ugly spectacle to behold, even if one does realize that mechanisms entirely beyond the patient's control are at work. A careful enquiry into what may have brought on such an attack almost invariably reveals that it is preceded by a strong unresolved sex-stimulation, the higher centers of the brain having blocked primitive diencephalic instinct gratification. The pressure is then let off through another primitive channel, which is oral gratification. In my experience the only thing that will cure this condition is uninhibited sex, a therapeutic procedure which is hardly ever feasible, for if it were, the patient would have adopted it without professional prompting, nor would this in any way correct the associated obesity. It would only raise new and often greater problems if used as a therapeutic measure.

Patients suffering from real compulsive eating are comparatively rare. In my practice they constitute about 1-2%. Treating them for obesity is a heartrending job. They do perfectly well between attacks, but a single bout occurring while under treatment may annul several weeks of therapy. Little wonder that such patients become discouraged. In these cases I have found that psychotherapy may make the patient fully understand the mechanism, but it does nothing to stop it. Perhaps society's growing sexual permissiveness will make compulsive eating even rarer.

Whether a patient is really suffering from compulsive eating or not is hard to decide before treatment because many obese patients think that their desire for food -- to them unmotivated -- is due to compulsive eating, while all the time it is merely a greater need for food. The only way to find out is to treat such patients. Those that suffer from real compulsive eating continue to have such attacks, while those who are not compulsive eaters never get an attack during treatment.

Reluctance to Lose Weight
Some patients are deeply attached to their fat and cannot bear the thought of losing it. If they are intelligent, popular and successful in spite of their handicap, this is a source of pride. Some fat girls look upon their condition as a safeguard against erotic involvements, of which they are afraid. They work out a pattern of life in which their obesity plays a determining role and then become reluctant to upset this pattern and face a new kind of life which will be entirely different after their figure has become normal and often very attractive. They fear that people will like them - or be jealous - on account of their figure rather than be attracted by their intelligence or character only. Some have a feeling that reducing means giving up an almost cherished and intimate part of themselves. In many of these cases psychotherapy can be helpful, as it enables these patients to see the whole situation in the full light of consciousness. An affectionate attachment to abnormal fat is usually seen in patients who became obese in childhood, but this is not necessarily so.

In all other cases the best psychotherapy can do in the usual treatment of obesity is to render the burden of hunger and never-ending dietary restrictions slightly more tolerable. Patients who
have successfully established an erotic transfer to their psychiatrist are often better able to bear their suffering as a secret labor of love.

There are thus a large number of ways in which obesity can be initiated, though the disorder itself is always due to the same mechanism, an inadequacy of the diencephalic fat-center and the laying down of abnormally fixed fat deposits in abnormal places. This means that once obesity has become established, it can no more be cured by eliminating those factors which brought it on than a fire can be extinguished by removing the cause of the conflagration. Thus a discussion of the various ways in which obesity can become established is useful from a preventative point of view, but it has no bearing on the treatment of the established condition. The elimination of factors which are clearly hastening the course of the disorder may slow down its progress or even halt it, but they can never correct it.

Not by Weight alone…

Weight alone is not a satisfactory criterion by which to judge whether a person is suffering from the disorder we call obesity or not. Every physician is familiar with the sylphlike lady who enters the consulting room and declares emphatically that she is getting horribly fat and wishes to reduce. Many an honest and sympathetic physician at once concludes that he is dealing with a "nut." If he is busy he will give her short shrift, but if he has time he will weigh her and show her tables to prove that she is actually underweight.

100

I have never yet seen or heard of such a lady being convinced by either procedure. The reason is that in my experience the lady is nearly always right and the doctor wrong. When such a patient is carefully examined one finds many signs of potential obesity, which is just about to become manifest as overweight. The patient distinctly feels that something is wrong with her, that a subtle change is taking place in her body, and this alarms her.

There are a number of signs and symptoms which are characteristic of obesity. In manifest obesity many and often all these signs and symptoms are present. In latent or just beginning cases some are always found, and it should be a rule that if two or more of the bodily signs are present, the case must be regarded as one that needs immediate help.

Signs and symptoms of obesity

The bodily signs may be divided into such as have developed before puberty, indicating a strong inherited factor, and those which develop at the onset of manifest disorder. Early signs are a disproportionately large size of the two upper front teeth, the first incisor, or a dimple on both sides of the sacral bone just above the buttocks. When the arms are outstretched with the palms upward, the forearms appear sharply angled outward from the upper arms. The same applies to the lower extremities. The patient cannot bring his feet together without the knees overlapping; he is, in fact, knock-kneed.

The beginning accumulation of abnormal fat shows as a little pad just below the nape of the neck, colloquially known as the Duchess' Hump. There is a triangular fatty bulge in front of the armpit when the arm is held against the body. When the skin is stretched by fat rapidly accumulating under it, it may split in the lower layers. When large and fresh, such tears are purple, but later they are transformed into white scar-tissue. Such striation, as it is called, commonly occurs on the abdomen of women during pregnancy, but in obesity it is frequently found on the breasts, the hips and occasionally on the shoulders. In many cases striation is so fine that the small white lines are only just visible. They are always a sure sign of obesity, and though this may be slight at the time of examination such patients can usually remember a period in their childhood when they were excessively chubby.
Another typical sign is a pad of fat on the insides of the knees, a spot where normal fat reserves are never stored. There may be a fold of skin over the pubic area and another fold may stretch round both sides of the chest, where a loose roll of fat can be picked up between two fingers. In the male an excessive accumulation of fat in the breasts is always indicative, while in the female the breast is usually, but not necessarily, large. Obviously excessive fat on the abdomen, the hips, thighs, upper arms, chin and shoulders are characteristic, and it is important to remember that any number of these signs may be present in persons whose weight is statistically normal; particularly if they are dieting on their own with iron determination.
Common clinical symptoms which are indicative only in their association and in the frame of the whole clinical picture are: frequent headaches, rheumatic pains without

detectable bony abnormality; a feeling of laziness and lethargy, often both physical and mental and frequently associated with insomnia, the patients saying that all they want is to rest; the frightening feeling of being famished and sometimes weak with hunger two to three hours after a hearty meal and an irresistible yearning for sweets and starchy food which often overcomes the patient quite suddenly and is sometimes substituted by a desire for alcohol; constipation and a spastic or irritable colon are unusually common among the obese, and so are menstrual disorders.

Returning once more to our sylphlike lady, we can say that a combination of some of these symptoms with a few of the typical bodily signs is sufficient evidence to take her case seriously. A human figure, male or female, can only be judged in the nude; any opinion based on the dressed appearance can be quite fantastically wide off the mark, and I feel myself driven to the conclusion that apart from frankly psychotic patients such as cases of anorexia nervosa; a morbid weight fixation does not exist. I have yet to see a patient who continues to complain after the figure has been rendered normal by adequate treatment.

The Emaciated Lady

I remember the case of a lady who was escorted into my consulting room while I was telephoning. She sat down in front of my desk, and when I looked up to greet her I saw the typical picture of advanced emaciation. Her dry skin hung loosely over the bones of her face, her neck was scrawny and collarbones and ribs stuck out from deep hollows. I immediately thought of cancer and decided to which of my colleagues at the hospital I would refer her. Indeed, I felt a little annoyed that my assistant had not explained to her that her case did not fall under my specialty. In answer to my query as to what I could do for her, she replied that she wanted to reduce. I tried to hide my surprise, but she must have noted a fleeting expression, for she smiled and said "I know that you think I'm mad, but just wait." With that she rose and came round to my side of the desk. Jutting out from a tiny waist she had enormous hips and thighs.

By using a technique which will presently be described, the abnormal fat on her hips was transferred to the rest of her body which had been emaciated by months of very severe dieting. At the end of a treatment lasting five weeks, she, a small woman, had lost 8 inches round her hips, while her face looked fresh and florid, the ribs were no longer visible and her weight was the same to the ounce as it had been at the first consultation.

Fat but not Obese

While a person who is statistically underweight may still be suffering from the disorder which causes obesity, it is also possible for a person to be statistically overweight without suffering from obesity. For such persons weight is no problem, as they can gain or lose at will and experience no difficulty in reducing their caloric intake. They are masters of their weight, which the obese are not. Moreover, their excess fat shows no preference for certain typical regions of the body, as does the fat in all cases of obesity. Thus, the decision whether a borderline case is really suffering from obesity or not cannot be made merely by consulting weight tables.

The Treatment Of Obesity

If obesity is always due to one very specific diencephalic deficiency, it follows that the only way to cure it is to correct this deficiency. At first this seemed an utterly hopeless undertaking. The greatest obstacle was that one could hardly hope to correct an inherited trait localized deep inside the brain, and while we did possess a number of drugs whose point of action was believed to be in the diencephalon, none of them had the slightest effect on the fat-center. There was not even a pointer showing a direction in which pharmacological research could move to find a drug that had such a specific action. The closest approach were the appetite-reducing drugs - the amphetamines----- but these cured nothing.

A Curious Observation

Mulling over this depressing situation, I remembered a rather curious observation made many years ago in India. At that time we knew very little about the function of the diencephalon, and my interest centered round the pituitary gland. Froehlich had described cases of extreme obesity and sexual underdevelopment in youths suffering from a new growth of the anterior pituitary lobe, producing what then became known as Froehlich's disease. However, it was very soon discovered that the identical syndrome, though running a less fulminating course, was quite common in patients whose pituitary gland was perfectly normal. These are the so-called "fat boys" with long, slender hands, breasts any flat-chested maiden would be proud to posses, large hips, buttocks and thighs with striation, knock-knees and underdeveloped genitals, often with undescended testicles.

It also became known that in these cases the sex organs could he developed by giving the patients injections of a substance extracted from the urine of pregnant women, it having been shown that when this substance was injected into sexually immature rats it made them precociously mature. The amount of substance which produced this effect in one rat was called one International Unit, and the purified extract was accordingly called "Human Chorionic Gonadotrophin" whereby chorionic signifies that it is produced in the placenta and gonadotropin that its action is sex gland directed.

The usual way of treating "fat boys" with underdeveloped genitals is to inject several hundred International Units twice a week. Human Chorionic Gonadotrophin which we shall henceforth simply call HCG is expensive and as "fat boys" are fairly common among Indians I tried to establish the smallest effective dose. In the course of this study three interesting things emerged. The first was that when fresh pregnancy-urine from the female ward was given in quantities of about 300 cc. by retention enema, as good results could be obtained as by injecting the pure substance. The second was that small daily doses appeared to be just as effective as much larger ones given twice a week. Thirdly, and that is the observation that concerns us here, when such patients were given small daily doses they seemed to lose their ravenous appetite though they neither gained nor lost weight. Strangely enough however, their shape did change. Though they were not restricted in diet, there was a distinct decrease in the circumference of their hips.

Fat on the Move

Remembering this, it occurred to me that the change in shape could only be explained by a movement of fat away from abnormal deposits on the hips, and if that were so there was just a chance that while such fat was in transition it might be available to the body as fuel. This was easy to find out, as in that case, fat on the move would be able to replace food. It should then he possible to keep a "fat boy" on a severely restricted diet without a feeling of hunger, in spite of a rapid loss of weight. When I tried this in typical cases of Froehlich's syndrome, I found that as long as such patients were given small daily doses of HCG they could comfortably go about their usual occupations on a diet of only 500 Calories daily and lose an average of about one pound per day. It was also perfectly evident that only abnormal fat was being consumed, as there were no signs of any depletion of normal fat. Their skin remained fresh and turgid, and gradually their figures became entirely normal, nor did the daily administration of HCG appear to have any side-effects other than beneficial.

From this point it was a small step to try the same method in all other forms of obesity. It took a few hundred cases to establish beyond reasonable doubt that the mechanism operates in exactly the same way and seemingly without exception in every case of obesity. I found that, though most patients were treated in the outpatients department, gross dietary errors rarely occurred. On the contrary, most patients complained that the two meals of 250 Calories each were more than they could manage, as they continually had a feeling of just having had a large meal.

Pregnancy and Obesity
Once this trail was opened, further observations seemed to fall into line. It is, for instance, well known that during pregnancy an obese woman can very easily lose weight. She can drastically reduce her diet without feeling hunger or discomfort and lose weight without in any way harming the child in her womb. It is also surprising to what extent a woman can suffer from pregnancy-vomiting without coming to any real harm.

Pregnancy is an obese woman's one great chance to reduce her excess weight. That she so rarely makes use of this opportunity is due to the erroneous notion, usually fostered by her elder relations, that she now has "two mouths to feed" and must "keep up her strength for the coming event. All modern obstetricians know that this is nonsense and that the more superfluous fat is lost the less difficult will be the confinement, though some still hesitate to prescribe a diet sufficiently low in Calories to bring about a drastic reduction.

A woman may gain weight during pregnancy, but she never becomes obese in the strict sense of the word. Under the influence of the HCG which circulates in enormous quantities in her body during pregnancy, her diencephalic banking capacity seems to be unlimited, and abnormal fixed deposits are never formed. At confinement she is suddenly deprived of HCG, and her diencephalic fat-center reverts to its normal capacity. It is only then that the abnormally accumulated fat is locked away again in a fixed deposit. From that moment on she is suffering from obesity and is subject to all its consequences.

Pregnancy seems to be the only normal human condition in which the diencephalic fat-banking capacity is unlimited. It is only during pregnancy that fixed fat deposits can be transferred back into the normal current account and freely drawn upon to make up for any nutritional deficit. During pregnancy, every ounce of reserve fat is placed at the disposal of the growing fetus. Were this not so, an obese woman, whose normal reserves are already depleted, would have the greatest difficulties in bringing her pregnancy to full term. There is considerable evidence to suggest that it is the HCG produced in large quantities in the placenta which brings about this diencephalic change.

Though we may be able to increase the dieneephalic fat banking capacity by injecting HCG, this does not in itself affect the weight, just as transferring monetary funds from a fixed deposit into a current account does not make a man any poorer; to become poorer it is also necessary that he freely spends the money which thus becomes available. In pregnancy the needs of the growing embryo take care of this to some extent, but in the treatment of obesity there is no embryo, and so a very severe dietary restriction must take its place for the duration of treatment.

Only when the fat which is in transit under the effect of HCG is actually consumed can more fat be withdrawn from the fixed deposits. In pregnancy it would be most undesirable if the fetus were offered ample food only when there is a high influx from the intestinal tract. Ideal nutritional conditions for the fetus can only be achieved when the mother's blood is continually saturated with food, regardless of whether she eats or not, as otherwise a period of starvation might hamper the steady growth of the embryo. It seems that HCG brings about this continual saturation of the blood, which is the reason why obese patients under treatment with HCG never feel hungry in spite of their drastically reduced food intake.

The Nature of Human Chorionic Gonadotropin

HCG is never found in the human body except during pregnancy and in those rare cases in which a residue of placental tissue continues to grow in the womb in what is known as a chorionic epithelioma. It is never found in the male. The human type of chorionic gonadotrophin is found only during the pregnancy of women and the great apes. It is produced in enormous quantities, so that during certain phases of her pregnancy a woman may excrete as much as one million International Units per day in her urine - enough to render a million infantile rats precociously mature. Other mammals make use of a different hormone, which can be extracted from their blood serum but not from their urine. Their placenta differs in this and other respects from that of man and the great apes. This animal chorionic gonadotrophin is much less rapidly broken down in the human body than HCG, and it is also less suitable for the treatment of obesity.

As often happens in medicine, much confusion has been caused by giving HCG its name before its true mode of action was understood. It has been explained that gonadotrophin literally means a sex-gland directed substance or hormone, and this is quite misleading. It dates from the early days when it was first found that HCG is able to render infantile sex glands mature, whereby it was entirely overlooked that it has no stimulating effect whatsoever on normally developed and normally functioning sex-glands. No amount of HCG is ever able to increase a normal sex function; it can only improve an abnormal one and in the young hasten the onset of puberty. However, this is no direct effect. HCG acts exclusively at a diencephalic level and there brings about a considerable increase in the functional capacity of all those centers which are working at maximum capacity.

The Real Gonadotrophins

Two hormones known in the female as follicle stimulating hormone (FSH) and corpus luteum stimulating hormone (LSH) are secreted by the anterior lobe of the pituitary gland. These hormones are real gonadotrophins because they directly govern the function of the ovaries. The anterior pituitary is in turn governed by the diencephalon, and so when there is an ovarian deficiency the diencephalic center concerned is hard put to correct matters by increasing the secretion from the anterior pituitary of FSH or LSH, as the case may be. When sexual deficiency is clinically present, this is a sign that the diencephalic center concerned is unable, in spite of maximal exertion, to cope with the demand for anterior pituitary stimulation. When then the administration of HCG increases the functional capacity of the diencephalon, all demands can be fully satisfied and the sex deficiency is corrected.

That this is the true mechanism underlying the presumed gonadotrophic action of HCG is confirmed by the fact that when the pituitary gland of infantile rats is removed before they are given HCG, the latter has no effect on their sex-glands. HCG cannot therefore have a direct sex gland stimulating action like that of the anterior pituitary gonadotrophins, as FSH and LSH are justly called. The latter are entirely different substances from that which can be extracted from pregnancy urine and which, unfortunately, is called chorionic gonadotrophin. It would be no more clumsy, and certainly far more appropriate, if HCG were henceforth called chorionic diencephalotrophin.

HCG no Sex Hormone

It cannot he sufficiently emphasized that HCG is not sex-hormone, that its action is identical in men, women, children and in those cases in which the sex-glands no longer function owing to old age or their surgical removal. The only sexual change it can bring

106

about after puberty is an improvement of a pre-existing deficiency, but never a stimulation beyond the normal. In an indirect way via the anterior pituitary, HCG regulates menstruation and facilitates conception, but it never virilizes a woman or feminizes a man. It neither makes men grow breasts nor does it interfere with their virility, though where this was deficient it may improve it. It never makes women grow a beard or develop a gruff voice. I have stressed this point only for the sake of my lay readers, because, it is our daily experience that when patients hear the word hormone they immediately jump to the conclusion that this must have something to do with the sex-sphere. They are not accustomed as we are, to think thyroid, insulin, cortisone, adrenalin etc, as hormones.

Importance and Potency of HCG

Owing to the fact that HCG has no direct action on any endocrine gland, its enormous importance in pregnancy has been overlooked and its potency underestimated. Though a pregnant woman can produce as much as one million units per day, we find that the injection of only 125 units per day is ample to reduce weight at the rate of roughly one pound per day, even in a colossus weighing 400 pounds, when associated with a 500-Calorie diet. It is no exaggeration to say that the flooding of the female body with HCG is by far the most spectacular hormonal event in pregnancy. It has an enormous protective importance for mother and child, and I even go so far as to say that no woman, and certainly not an obese one, could carry her pregnancy to term without it.

If I can be forgiven for comparing my fellow-endocrinologists with wicked Godmothers, HCG has certainly been their Cinderella, and I can only romantically hope that its extraordinary effect on abnormal fat will prove to be its Fairy Godmother.

HCG has been known for over half a century. It is the substance which Aschheim and Zondek so brilliantly used to diagnose early pregnancy out of the urine. Apart from that, the only thing it did in the experimental laboratory was to produce precocious rats, and that was not particularly stimulating to further research at a time when much more thrilling endocrinological discoveries were pouring in from all sides, sweeping, HCG into the stiller back waters.

Complicating Disorders

Some complicating disorders are often associated with obesity, and these we must briefly discuss. The most important associated disorders and the ones in which obesity seems to play a precipitating or at least an aggravating role are the following: the stable type of diabetes, gout, rheumatism and arthritis, high blood pressure and hardening of the arteries, coronary disease and cerebral hemorrhage.

Apart from the fact that they are often - though not necessarily - associated with obesity, these disorders have two things in common. In all of them, modern research is becoming more and more inclined to believe that diencephalic regulations play a dominant role in their causation. The other common factor is that they either improve or do not occur during pregnancy. In the latter respect they are joined by many other disorders not necessarily associated with obesity. Such disorders are, for instance, colitis, duodenal or gastric ulcers, certain allergies, psoriasis, loss of hair, brittle fingernails, migraine, etc.

If HCG + diet does in the obese bring about those diencephalic changes which are characteristic of pregnancy, one would expect to see an improvement in all these conditions comparable to that seen in real pregnancy. The administration of HCG does in fact do this in a remarkable way.

Diabetes

In an obese patient suffering from a fairly advanced case of stable diabetes of many years duration in which the blood sugar may range from 3-400 mg%, it is often possible to stop all antidiabetic medication after the first few days of treatment. The blood sugar continues to drop from day to day and often reaches normal values in 2-3 weeks. As in pregnancy, this phenomenon is not observed in the brittle type of diabetes, and as some cases that are predominantly stable may have a small brittle factor in their clinical makeup, all obese diabetics have to be kept under a very careful and expert watch.

A brittle case of diabetes is primarily due to the inability of the pancreas to produce sufficient insulin, while in the stable type, diencephalic regulations seem to be of greater importance. That is possibly the reason why the stable form responds so well to the HCG method of treating obesity, whereas the brittle type does not. Obese patients are generally suffering from the stable type, but a stable type may gradually change into a brittle one, which is usually associated with a loss of weight. Thus, when an obese diabetic finds that he is losing weight without diet or treatment, he should at once have his diabetes expertly attended to. There is some evidence to suggest that the change from stable to brittle is more liable to occur in patients who are taking insulin for their stable diabetes.

Rheumatism

All rheumatic pains, even those associated with demonstrable bony lesions, improve subjectively within a few days of treatment, and often require neither cortisone nor salicylates. Again this is a well known phenomenon in pregnancy, and while under treatment with HCG + diet the effect is no less dramatic. As it does after pregnancy, the pain of deformed joints returns after treatment, but smaller doses of pain-relieving drugs seem able to control it satisfactorily after weight reduction. In any case, the HCG method makes it possible in obese arthritic patients to interrupt prolonged cortisone treatment without a recurrence of pain. This in itself is most welcome, but there is the added advantage that the treatment stimulates the secretion of ACTH in a physiological manner and that this regenerates the adrenal cortex, which is apt to suffer under prolonged cortisone treatment.

Cholesterol

The exact extent to which the blood cholesterol is involved in hardening of the arteries, high blood pressure and coronary disease is not as yet known, but it is now widely admitted that the blood cholesterol level is governed by diencephalic mechanisms. The behavior of circulating cholesterol is therefore of particular interest during the treatment of obesity with HCG. Cholesterol circulates in two forms, which we call free and esterified. Normally these fractions are present in a proportion of about 25% free to 75% esterified cholesterol, and it is the latter fraction which damages the walls of the arteries. In pregnancy this proportion is reversed and it may he taken for granted that arteriosclerosis never gets worse during pregnancy for this very reason.

To my knowledge, the only other condition in which the proportion of free to esterified cholesterol is reversed is during the treatment of obesity with HCG + diet, when exactly the same phenomenon takes place. This seems an important indication of how closely a patient under HCG treatment resembles a pregnant woman in diencephalic behavior.

When the total amount of circulating cholesterol is normal before treatment, this absolute amount is neither significantly increased nor decreased. But when an obese patient with an abnormally high cholesterol and already showing signs of arteriosclerosis is treated with HCG, his blood pressure drops and his coronary circulation seems to improve, and yet his total blood cholesterol may soar to heights never before reached.

At first this greatly alarmed us. But then we saw that the patients came to no harm even if treatment was continued and we found in follow-up examinations undertaken some months after treatment that the cholesterol was much better than it had been before treatment. As the increase is mostly in the form of the not dangerous free cholesterol, we gradually came to welcome the phenomenon. Today we believe that the rise is entirely due to the liberation of recent cholesterol deposits that have not yet undergone calcification in the arterial wall and therefore highly beneficial.

Gout

An identical behavior is found in the blood uric acid level of patients suffering from gout. Predictably such patients get an acute and often severe attack after the first few days of HCG treatment but then remain entirely free of pain, in spite of the fact that their blood uric acid often shows a marked increase which may persist for several months after treatment. Those patients who have regained their normal weight remain free of symptoms regardless of what they eat, while those that require a second course of treatment get another attack of gout as soon as the second course is initiated. We do not yet know what diencephalic mechanisms are involved in gout; possibly emotional factors play a role, and it is worth remembering that the disease does not occur in women of childbearing age. We now give 2 tablets daily of ZYLORIC to all patients who give a history of gout and have a high blood uric acid level. In this way we can completely avoid attacks during treatment.

Blood Pressure

Patients who have brought themselves to the brink of malnutrition by exaggerated dieting, laxatives etc, often have an abnormally low blood pressure. In these cases the blood pressure rises to normal values at the beginning of treatment and then very gradually drops, as it always does in patients with a normal blood pressure. Normal values are always regained a few days after the treatment is over. Of this lowering of the blood pressure during treatment the patients are not aware. When the blood pressure is abnormally high, and provided there are no detectable renal lesions, the pressure drops, as it usually does in pregnancy. The drop is often very rapid, so rapid in fact that it sometimes is advisable to slow down the process with pressure sustaining medication until the circulation has had a few days time to adjust itself to the new situation. On the other hand, among the thousands of cases treated, we have never seen any untoward incident which could be attributed to the rather sudden drop in high blood pressure.

When a woman suffering from high blood pressure becomes pregnant her blood pressure very soon drops, but after her confinement it may gradually rise back to its former level. Similarly, a high blood pressure present before HCG treatment tends to rise again after the treatment is over, though this is not always the case. But the former high levels are rarely reached, and we have gathered the impression that such relapses respond better to orthodox drugs such as Reserpine than before treatment.

Peptic Ulcers

In our cases of obesity with gastric or duodenal ulcers we have noticed a surprising subjective improvement in spite of a diet which would generally be considered most inappropriate for an ulcer patient. Here, too, there is a similarity with pregnancy, in which peptic ulcers hardly ever occur. However we have seen two cases with a previous history of several hemorrhages in which a bleeding occurred within 2 weeks of the end of treatment.

Psoriasis, Fingernails, Hair, Varicose Ulcers

 As in pregnancy, psoriasis greatly improves during treatment but may relapse when the treatment is over. Most patients spontaneously report a marked improvement in the condition of brittle fingernails. The loss of hair not infrequently associated with obesity is temporarily arrested, though in very rare cases an increased loss of hair has been reported. I remember a case in which a patient developed a patchy baldness - so called alopecia areata - after a severe emotional shock, just before she was about to start an HCG treatment. Our dermatologist diagnosed the case as a particularly severe one, predicting that all the hair would be lost. He counseled against the reducing treatment, but in view of my previous experience and as the patient was very anxious not to postpone reducing, I discussed the matter with the dermatologist and it was agreed that, having fully acquainted the patient with the situation, the treatment should be started. During the treatment, which lasted four weeks, the further development of the bald patches was almost, if not quite, arrested; however, within a week of having finished the course of HCG, all the remaining hair fell out as predicted by the dermatologist. The interesting point is that the treatment was able to postpone this result but not to prevent it. The patient has now grown a new shock of hair of which she is justly proud.

In obese patients with large varicose ulcers we were surprised to find that these ulcers heal rapidly under treatment with HCG. We have since treated non obese patients suffering from varicose ulcers with daily injections of HCG on normal diet with equally good results.

The "Pregnant" Male

When a male patient hears that he is about to be put into a condition which in some respects resembles pregnancy, he is usually shocked and horrified. The physician must therefore carefully explain that this does not mean that he will be feminized and that HCG in no way interferes with his sex. He must be made to understand that in the interest of the propagation of the species nature provides for a perfect functioning of the regulatory headquarters in the diencephalon during pregnancy and that we are merely using this natural safeguard as a means of correcting the diencephalic disorder which is responsible for his overweight.

TECHNIQUE

Warnings

I must warn the lay reader that what follows is mainly for the treating physician and most certainly not a do-it-yourself primer. Many of the expressions used mean something entirely different to a qualified doctor than that which their common use implies, and only a physician can correctly interpret the symptoms which may arise during treatment. Any patient who thinks he can reduce by taking a few "shots" and eating less is not only sure to be disappointed but may be heading for serious trouble. The benefit the patient can derive from reading this part of the book is a fuller realization of how very important it is for him to follow to the letter his physician's instructions.

In treating obesity with the HCG + diet method we are handling what is perhaps the most complex organ in the human body. The diencephalon's functional equilibrium is delicately poised, so that whatever happens in one part has repercussions in others. In obesity this balance is out of kilter and can only be restored if the technique I am about to describe is followed implicitly. Even seemingly insignificant deviations, particularly those that at first sight seem to be an improvement, are very liable to produce most disappointing results and even annul the effect completely. For instance, if the diet is increased from 500 to 600 or 700 Calories, the loss of weight is quite unsatisfactory. If the daily dose of HCG is raised to 200 or more units daily its action often appears to be reversed, possibly because larger doses evoke diencephalic counter-regulations. On the other hand, the diencephalon is an extremely robust organ in spite of its unbelievable intricacy. From an evolutionary point of view it is one of the oldest organs in our body and its evolutionary history dates back more than 500 million years. This has tendered it extraordinarily adaptable to all natural exigencies, and that is one of the main reasons why the human species was able to evolve. What its evolution did not prepare it for were the conditions to which human culture and civilization now expose it.

History taking

When a patient first presents himself for treatment, we take a general history and note the time when the first signs of overweight were observed. We try to establish the highest weight the patient has ever had in his life (obviously excluding pregnancy), when this was, and what measures have hitherto been taken in an effort to reduce.

It has been our experience that those patients who have been taking thyroid preparations for long periods have a slightly lower average loss of weight under treatment with HCG than those who have never taken thyroid. This is even so in those patients who have been taking thyroid because they had an abnormally low basal metabolic rate. In many of these cases the low BMR is not due to any intrinsic deficiency of the thyroid gland, but rather to a lack of diencephalic stimulation of the thyroid gland via the anterior pituitary lobe. We never allow thyroid to be taken during treatment, and yet a BMR which was very low before treatment is usually found to be normal after a week or two of HCG + diet. Needless to say, this does not apply to those cases in which a thyroid deficiency has been produced by the surgical removal of a part of an overactive gland. It is also most important to ascertain whether the patient has taken diuretics (water eliminating pills) as this also decreases the weight loss under the HCG regimen.

Returning to our procedure, we next ask the patient a few questions to which he is held to reply simply with "yes" or "no". These questions are: Do you suffer from headaches? rheumatic pains? menstrual disorders? constipation? breathlessness or exertion? swollen ankles? Do you consider yourself greedy? Do you feel the need to eat snacks between meals?

The patient then strips and is weighed and measured. The normal weight for his height, age, skeletal and muscular build is established from tables of statistical averages, whereby in women it is often necessary to make an allowance for particularly large and heavy breasts. The degree of overweight is then calculated, and from this the duration of treatment can be roughly assessed on the basis of an average loss of weight of a little less than a pound, say 300-400 grams-per injection, per day. It is a particularly interesting feature of the HCG treatment that in reasonably cooperative patients this figure is remarkably constant, regardless of sex, age and degree of overweight.

The Duration of Treatment

Patients who need to lose 15 pounds (7 kg.) or less require 26 days treatment with 23 daily injections. The extra three days are needed because all patients must continue the 500-Calorie diet for three days after the last injection. This is a very essential part of the treatment, because if they start eating normally as long as there is even a trace of HCG in their body they put on weight alarmingly at the end of the treatment. After three days when all the HCG has been eliminated this does not happen, because the blood is then no longer saturated with food and can thus accommodate an extra influx from the intestines without increasing its volume by retaining water.

We never give a treatment lasting less than 26 days, even in patients needing to lose only 5 pounds. It seems that even in the mildest cases of obesity the diencephalon requires about three weeks rest from the maximal exertion to which it has been previously subjected in order to regain fully its normal fat-banking capacity. Clinically this expresses itself, in the fact that, when in these mild cases, treatment is stopped as soon as the weight is normal, which may be achieved in a week, it is much more easily regained than after a full course of 23 injections.

As soon as such patients have lost all their abnormal superfluous fat, they at once begin to feel ravenously hungry in spite of continued injections. This is because HCG only puts abnormal fat into circulation and cannot, in the doses used, liberate normal fat deposits; indeed, it seems to prevent their consumption. As soon as their statistically normal weight is reached, these patients are put on 800-1000 Calories for the rest of the treatment.

The diet is arranged in such a way that the weight remains perfectly stationary and is thus continued for three days after the 23rd injection. Only then are the patients free to eat anything they please except sugar and starches for the next three weeks.

Such early cases are common among actresses, models, and persons who are tired of obesity, having seen its ravages in other members of their family. Film actresses frequently explain that they must weigh less than normal. With this request we flatly refuse to comply, first, because we undertake to cure a disorder, not to create a new one, and second, because it is in the nature of the HCG method that it is self limiting. It becomes completely ineffective as soon as all abnormal fat is consumed. Actresses with a slight tendency to obesity, having tried all manner of reducing methods, invariably come to the conclusion that their figure is satisfactory only when they are underweight, simply because none of these methods remove their superfluous fat deposits. When they see that under HCG their figure improves out of all proportion to the amount of weight lost, they are nearly always content to remain within their normal weight-range.

When a patient has more than 15 pounds to lose the treatment takes longer but the maximum we give in a single course is 40 injections, nor do we as a rule allow patients to lose more than 34 lbs. (15 Kg.) at a time. The treatment is stopped when either 34 lbs. have been lost or 40 injections have been given. The only exception we make is in the case of grotesquely obese patients who may be allowed to lose an additional 5-6 lbs. if this occurs before the 40 injections are up.

Immunity to HCG

The reason for limiting a course to 40 injections is that by then some patients may begin to show signs of HCG immunity. Though this phenomenon is well known, we cannot as yet define the underlying mechanism. Maybe after a certain length of time the body learns to break down and eliminate HCG very rapidly, or possibly prolonged treatment leads to some sort of counter-regulation which annuls the diencephalic effect.

After 40 daily injections it takes about six weeks before this so called immunity is lost and HCG again becomes fully effective. Usually after about 40 injections patients may feel the onset of immunity as hunger which was previously absent. In those comparatively rare cases in which signs of immunity develop before the full course of 40 injections has been completed-say at the 35th injection- treatment must be stopped at once, because if it is continued the patients begin to look weary and drawn, feel weak and hungry and any further loss of weight achieved is then always at the expense of normal fat. This is not only undesirable, but normal fat is also instantly regained as soon as the patient is returned to a free diet.

Patients who need only 23 injections may be injected daily, including Sundays, as they never develop immunity. In those that take 40 injections the onset of immunity can be delayed if they are given only six injections a week, leaving out Sundays or any other day they choose, provided that it is always the same day. On the days on which they do not receive the injections they usually feel a slight sensation of hunger. At first we thought that this might be purely psychological, but we found that when normal saline is injected without the patient's knowledge the same phenomenon occurs.

Menstruation

During menstruation no injections are given, but the diet is continued and causes no hardship; yet as soon as the menstruation is over, the patients become extremely hungry unless the injections are resumed at once. It is very impressive to see the suffering of a woman who has continued her diet for a day or two beyond the end of the period without coming for her injection and then to hear the next day that all hunger ceased within a few hours after the injection and to see her once again content, florid and cheerful. While on the question of menstruation it must he added that in teenaged girls the period may in some rare cases be delayed and exceptionally stop altogether. If then later this is artificially induced some weight may be regained.

Further Courses

Patients requiring the loss of more than 34 lbs. must have a second or even more courses. A second course can be started after an interval of not less than six weeks, though the pause can be more than six weeks. When a third, fourth or even fifth course is necessary, the interval between courses should be made progressively longer. Between a second and third course eight weeks should elapse, between a third and fourth course twelve weeks, between a fourth and fifth course twenty weeks and between a fifth and sixth course six months. In this way it is possible to bring about a weight reduction of 100 lbs. and more if required without the least hardship to the patient.

114

In general, men do slightly better than women and often reach a somewhat higher average daily loss. Very advanced cases do a little better than early ones, but it is a remarkable fact that this difference is only just statistically significant.

Conditions that must be accepted before treatment

On the basis of these data the probable duration of treatment can he calculated with considerable accuracy, and this is explained to the patient. It is made clear to him that during the course of treatment he must attend the clinic daily to be weighed, injected and generally checked. All patients that live in Rome or have resident friends or relations with whom they can stay are treated as out-patients, but patients coming from abroad must stay in the hospital, as no hotel or restaurant can be relied upon to prepare the diet with sufficient accuracy. These patients have their meals, sleep, and attend the clinic in the hospital, but are otherwise free to spend their time as they please in the city and its surroundings sightseeing, bathing or theater-going.

It is also made clear that between courses the patient gets no treatment and is free to eat anything he pleases except starches and sugar during the first 3 weeks. It is impressed upon him that he will have to follow the prescribed diet to the letter and that after the first three days this will cost him no effort, as he will feel no hunger and may indeed have difficulty in getting down the 500 Calories which he will be given. If these conditions are not acceptable the case is refused, as any compromise or half measure is bound to prove utterly disappointing to patient and physician alike and is a waste of time and energy.

Though a patient can only consider himself really cured when he has been reduced to his statistically normal weight, we do not insist that he commit himself to that extent. Even a partial loss of overweight is highly beneficial, and it is our experience that once a patient has completed a first course he is so enthusiastic about the ease with which the - to him surprising - results are achieved that he almost invariably comes back for more. There certainly can be no doubt that in my clinic more time is spent on damping over-enthusiasm than on insisting that the rules of the treatment be observed.

Examining the patient

Only when agreement is reached on the points so far discussed do we proceed with the examination of the patient. A note is made of the size of the first upper incisor, of a pad of fat on the nape of the neck, at the axilla and on the inside of the knees. The presence of striation, a suprapubic fold, a thoracic fold, angulation of elbow and knee joint, breast-development in men and women, edema of the ankles and the state of genital development in the male are noted.

Wherever this seems indicated we X-ray the sella turcica, as the bony capsule which contains the pituitary gland is called, measure the basal metabolic rate, X-ray the chest and take an electrocardiogram. We do a blood-count and a sedimentation rate and estimate uric acid, cholesterol, iodine and sugar in the fasting blood.

Gain before Loss

Patients whose general condition is low, owing to excessive previous dieting, must eat to capacity for about one week before starting treatment, regardless of how much weight they may gain in the process. One cannot keep a patient comfortably on 500 Calories unless his normal fat reserves are reasonably well stocked. It is for this reason also that every case, even those that are actually gaining must eat to capacity of the most fattening food they can get down until they have had the third injection. It is a fundamental mistake to put a patient on 500 Calories as soon as the injections are started, as it seems to take about three injections before abnormally deposited fat begins to circulate and thus become available.

We distinguish between the first three injections, which we call "non-effective" as far as the loss of weight is concerned, and the subsequent injections given while the patient is dieting, which we call "effective". The average loss of weight is calculated on the number of effective injections and from the weight reached on the day of the third injection which may be well above what it was two days earlier when the first injection was given.

Most patients who have been struggling with diets for years and know how rapidly they gain if they let themselves go are very hard to convince of the absolute necessity of gorging for at least two days, and yet this must he insisted upon categorically if the further course of treatment is to run smoothly. Those patients who have to be put on forced feeding for a week before starting the injections usually gain weight rapidly - four to six pounds in 24 hours is not unusual - but after a day or two this rapid gain generally levels off. In any case, the whole gain is usually lost in the first 48 hours of dieting. It is necessary to proceed in this manner because the gain re-stocks the depleted normal reserves, whereas the subsequent loss is from the abnormal deposits only.

Patients in a satisfactory general condition and those who have not just previously restricted their diet start forced feeding on the day of the first injection. Some patents say that they can no longer overeat because their stomach has shrunk after years of restrictions. While we know that no stomach ever shrinks, we compromise by insisting that they eat frequently of highly concentrated foods such as milk chocolate, pastries with whipped cream sugar, fried meats (particularly pork), eggs and bacon, mayonnaise, bread with thick butter and jam, etc. The time and trouble spent on pressing this point upon incredulous or reluctant patients is always amply rewarded afterwards by the complete absence of those difficulties which patients who have disregarded these instructions are liable to experience.

During the two days of forced feeding from the first to the third injection - many patients are surprised that contrary to their previous experience they do not gain weight and some even lose. The explanation is that in these cases there is a compensatory flow of urine, which drains excessive water from the body. To some extent this seems to be a direct action of HCG, but it may also be due to a higher protein intake, as we know that a protein-deficient diet makes the body retain water.

Starting treatment

In menstruating women, the best time to start treatment is immediately after a period. Treatment may also be started later, but it is advisable to have at least ten days in hand before the onset of the next period. Similarly, the end of a course of HCG should never be made to coincide with menstruation. If things should happen to work out that way, it is better to give the last injection three days before the expected date of the menses so that a normal diet can he resumed at onset. Alternatively, at least three injections should be given after the period, followed by the usual three days of dieting. This rule need not be observed in such patients who have reached their normal weight before the end of treatment and are already on a higher caloric diet.

Patients who require more than the minimum of 23 injections and who therefore skip one day a week in order to postpone immunity to HCG cannot have their third injections on the day before the interval. Thus if it is decided to skip Sundays, the treatment can be started on any day of the week except Thursdays. Supposing they start on Thursday, they will have their third injection on Saturday, which is also the day on which they start their 500 Calorie diet. They would then have no injection on the second day of dieting; this exposes them to an unnecessary hardship, as without the injection they will feel particularly hungry. Of course, the difficulty can be overcome by exceptionally injecting them on the first Sunday. If this day falls between the first and second or between the second and third injection, we usually prefer to give the patient the extra day of forced feeding, which the majority rapturously enjoy.

The Diet

The 500 Calorie diet is explained on the day of the second injection to those patients who will be preparing their own food, and it is most important that the person who will actually cook is present - the wife, the mother or the cook, as the case may be. Here in Italy patients are given the following diet sheet.

Breakfast:	Tea or coffee in any quantity without sugar. Only one tablespoonful of milk allowed in 24 hours. Saccharin or Stevia may be used.
Lunch:	1. 100 grams of veal, beef, chicken breast, fresh white fish, lobster, crab, or shrimp. All visible fat must be carefully removed before cooking, and the meat must be weighed raw. It must be boiled or grilled without additional fat. Salmon, eel, tuna, herring, dried or pickled fish are not allowed. The chicken breast must be removed from the bird.
	2. One type of vegetable only to be chosen from the following: spinach, chard, chicory, beet-greens, green salad, tomatoes, celery, fennel, onions, red radishes, cucumbers, asparagus, cabbage.
	3. One breadstick (grissino) or one Melba toast.
	4. An apple, orange, or a handful of strawberries or one-half grapefruit.
Dinner :	The same four choices as lunch (above.)

The juice of one lemon daily is allowed for all purposes. Salt, pepper, vinegar, mustard powder, garlic, sweet basil, parsley, thyme, majoram, etc., may be used for seasoning, but no oil, butter or dressing.

Tea, coffee, plain water, or mineral water are the only drinks allowed, but they may be taken in any quantity and at all times.

In fact, the patient should drink about 2 liters of these fluids per day. Many patients are afraid to drink so much because they fear that this may make them retain more water. This is a wrong notion as the body is more inclined to store water when the intake falls below its normal requirements.

The fruit or the breadstick may be eaten between meals instead of with lunch or dinner, but not more than than four items listed for lunch and dinner may be eaten at one meal.

No medicines or cosmetics other than lipstick, eyebrow pencil and powder may be used without special permission.

Every item in the list is gone over carefully, continually stressing the point that no variations other than those listed may be introduced. All things not listed are forbidden, and the patient is assured that nothing permissible has been left out. The 100 grams of meat must he scrupulously weighed raw after all visible fat has been removed. To do this accurately the patient must have a letter-scale, as kitchen scales are not sufficiently accurate and the butcher should certainly not be relied upon. Those not uncommon patients who feel that even so little food is too much for them, can omit anything they wish.

There is no objection to breaking up the two meals. For instance having a breadstick and an apple for breakfast or an orange before going to bed, provided they are deducted from the regular meals. The whole daily ration of two breadsticks or two fruits may not be eaten at the same time, nor can any item saved from the previous day be added on the following day. In the beginning patients are advised to check every meal against their diet sheet before starting to eat and not to rely on their memory. It is also worth pointing out that any attempt to observe this diet without HCG will lead to trouble in two to three days. We have had cases in which patients have proudly flaunted their dieting powers in front of their friends without mentioning the fact that they are also receiving treatment with HCG. They let their friends try the same diet, and when this proves to be a failure - as it necessarily must - the patient starts raking in unmerited kudos for superhuman willpower.

It should also be mentioned that two small apples weighing as much as one large one never the less have a higher caloric value and are therefore not allowed though there is no restriction on the size of one apple. Some people do not realize that a tangerine is not an orange and that chicken breast does not mean the breast of any other fowl, nor does it mean a wing or drumstick.

The most tiresome patients are those who start counting Calories and then come up with all manner of ingenious variations which they compile from their little books. When one has spent years of weary research trying to make a diet as attractive as possible without jeopardizing the loss of weight, culinary geniuses who are out to improve their unhappy lot are hard to take.

Making up the Calories

The diet used in conjunction with HCG must not exceed 500 Calories per day, and the way these Calories are made up is of utmost importance. For instance, if a patient drops the apple and eats an extra breadstick instead, he will not be getting more Calories but he will not lose weight. There are a number of foods, particularly fruits and vegetables, which have the same or even lower caloric values than those listed as permissible, and yet we find that they interfere with the regular loss of weight under HCG, presumably owing to the nature of their composition. Pimiento peppers, okra, artichokes and pears are examples of this.

While this diet works satisfactorily in Italy, certain modifications have to be made in other countries. For instance, American beef has almost double the caloric value of South Italian beef, which is not marbled with fat. This marbling is impossible to remove. In America, therefore, low-grade veal should be used for one meal and fish (excluding all those species such as herring, mackerel, tuna, salmon, eel, etc., which have a high fat content, and all dried, smoked or pickled fish), chicken breast, lobster, crawfish, prawns, shrimps, crabmeat or kidneys for the other meal. Where the Italian breadsticks, the so-called grissini, are not available, one Melba toast may be used instead, though they are psychologically less satisfying. A Melba toast has about the same weight as the very porous grissini which is much more to look at and to chew.

In many countries specially prepared unsweetened and low Calorie foods are freely available, and some of these can be tentatively used. When local conditions or the feeding habits of the population make changes necessary it must be borne in mind that the total daily intake must not exceed 500 Calories if the best possible results are to be obtained, that the daily ration should contain 200 grams of fat-free protein and a very small amount of starch.

Just as the daily dose of HCG is the same in all cases, so the same diet proves to be satisfactory for a small elderly lady of leisure or a hard working muscular giant. Under the effect of HCG the obese body is always able to obtain all the Calories it needs from the abnormal fat deposits, regardless of whether it uses up 1500 or 4000 per day. It must be made very clear to the patient that he is living to a far greater extent on the fat which he is losing than on what he eats.

Many patients ask why eggs are not allowed. The contents of two good sized eggs are roughly equivalent to 100 grams of meat, but fortunately the yolk contains a large amount of fat, which is undesirable. Very occasionally we allow egg - boiled, poached or raw - to patients who develop an aversion to meat, but in this case they must add the white of three eggs to the one they eat whole. In countries where cottage cheese made from skimmed milk is available 100 grams may occasionally be used instead of the meat, but no other cheeses are allowed.

Vegetarians

Strict vegetarians such as orthodox Hindus present a special problem, because milk and curds are the only animal protein they will eat. To supply them with sufficient protein of animal origin they must drink 500 cc. of skimmed milk per day, though part of this ration can be taken as curds. As far as fruit, vegetables and starch are concerned, their diet is the same as that of non-vegetarians; they cannot be allowed their usual intake of vegetable proteins from leguminous plants such as beans or from wheat or nuts, nor can they have their customary rice. In spite of these severe restrictions, their average loss is about half that of non-vegetarians, presumably owing to the sugar content of the milk.

Faulty Dieting

Few patients will take one's word for it that the slightest deviation from the diet has under HCG disastrous results as far as the weight is concerned. This extreme sensitivity has the advantage that the smallest error is immediately detectable at the daily weighing but most patients have to make the experience before they will believe it.

Persons in high official positions such as embassy personnel, politicians, senior executives, etc., who are obliged to attend social functions to which they cannot bring their meager meal must be told beforehand that an official dinner will cost them the loss of about three days treatment, however careful they are and in spite of a friendly and would-be cooperative host. We generally advise them to avoid all-round embarrassment, the almost inevitable turn of conversation to their weight problem and the outpouring of lay counsel from their table partners by not letting it be known that they are under treatment. They should take dainty servings of everything, hide what they can under the cutlery and book the gain which may take three days to get rid of as one of the sacrifices which their profession entails. Allowing three days for their correction, such incidents do not jeopardize the treatment, provided they do not occur all too frequently in which case treatment should be postponed to a socially more peaceful season.

Vitamins and Anemia

Sooner or later most patients express a fear that they may be running out of vitamins or that the restricted diet may make them anemic. On this score the physician can confidently relieve their apprehension by explaining that every time they lose a pound of fatty tissue, which they do almost daily, only the actual fat is burned up; all the vitamins, the proteins, the blood, and the minerals which this tissue contains in abundance are fed back into the body. Actually, a low blood count not due to any serious disorder of the blood forming tissues improves during treatment, and we have never encountered a significant protein deficiency nor signs of a lack of vitamins in patients who are dieting regularly.

The First Days of Treatment

On the day of the third injection it is almost routine to hear two remarks. One is: "You know, Doctor, I'm sure it's only psychological, but I already feel quite different". So common is this remark, even from very skeptical patients that we hesitate to accept the psychological interpretation. The other typical remark is: "Now that I have been allowed to eat anything I want, I can't get it down. Since yesterday I feel like a stuffed pig. Food just doesn't seem to interest me any more, and I am longing to get on with your diet". Many patients notice that they are passing more urine and that the swelling in their ankles is less even before they start dieting.

On the day of the fourth injection most patients declare that they are feeling fine. They have usually lost two pounds or more, some say they feel a bit empty but hasten to explain that this does not amount to hunger. Some complain of a mild headache of which they have been forewarned and for which they have been given permission to take aspirin.

During the second and third day of dieting - that is, the fifth and sixth injection-these minor complaints improve while the weight continues to drop at about double the usually overall average of almost one pound per day, so that a moderately severe case may by the fourth day of dieting have lost as much as 8- 10 lbs.

It is usually at this point that a difference appears between those patients who have literally eaten to capacity during the first two days of treatment and those who have not. The former feel remarkably well; they have no hunger, nor do they feel tempted when others eat normally at the same table. They feel lighter, more clear-headed and notice a desire to move quite contrary to their previous lethargy. Those who have disregarded the advice to eat to capacity continue to have minor discomforts and do not have the same euphoric sense of well-being until about a week later. It seems that their normal fat reserves require that much more time before they are fully stocked.

Fluctuations in weight loss
After the fourth or fifth day of dieting the daily loss of weight begins to decrease to one pound or somewhat less per day, and there is a smaller urinary output. Men often continue to lose regularly at that rate, but women are more irregular in spite of faultless dieting. There may be no drop at all for two or three days and then a sudden loss which reestablishes the normal average. These fluctuations are entirely due to variations in the retention and elimination of water, which are more marked in women than in men.

The weight registered by the scale is determined by two processes not necessarily synchronized. Under the influence of HCG, fat is being extracted from the cells, in which it is stored in the fatty tissue. When these cells are empty and therefore serve no purpose, the body breaks down the cellular structure and absorbs it, but breaking up of useless cells, connective tissue, blood vessels, etc., may lag behind the process of fat-extraction. When this happens the body appears to replace some of the extracted fat with water which is retained for this purpose. As water is heavier than fat the scales may show no loss of weight, although sufficient fat has actually been consumed to make up for the deficit in the 500-Calorie diet. When then such tissue is finally broken down, the water is liberated and there is a sudden flood of urine and a marked loss of weight. This simple interpretation of what is really an extremely complex mechanism is the one we give those patients who want to know why it is that on certain days they do not lose, though they have committed no dietary error.

Patients who have previously regularly used diuretics as a method of reducing, lose fat during the first two or three weeks of treatment which shows in their measurements, but the scale may show little or no loss because they are replacing the normal water content of their body which has been dehydrated. Diuretics should never be used for reducing.

Interruptions of Weight Loss

We distinguish four types of interruption in the regular daily loss. The first is the one that has already been mentioned in which the weight stays stationary for a day or two, and this occurs, particularly towards the end of a course, in almost every case.

The Plateau

The second type of interruption we call a "plateau". A plateau lasts 4-6 days and frequently occurs during the second half of a full course, particularly in patients that have been doing well and whose overall average of nearly a pound per effective injection has been maintained. Those who are losing more than the average all have a plateau sooner or later. A plateau always corrects, itself, but many patients who have become accustomed to a regular daily loss get unnecessarily worried and begin to fret. No amount of explanation convinces them that a plateau does not mean that they are no longer responding normally to treatment.

In such cases we consider it permissible, for purely psychological reasons, to break up the plateau. This can be done in two ways. One is a so-called "apple day". An apple-day begins at lunch and continues until just before lunch of the following day. The patients are given six large apples and are told to eat one whenever they feel the desire though six apples is the maximum allowed. During an apple-day no other food or liquids except plain water are allowed and of water they may only drink just enough to quench an uncomfortable thirst if eating an apple still leaves them thirsty. Most patients feel no need for water and are quite happy with their six apples. Needless to say, an apple-day may never be given on the day on which there is no injection. The apple-day produces a gratifying loss of weight on the following day, chiefly due to the elimination of water. This water is not regained when the patients resume their normal 500-Calorie diet at lunch, and on the following days they continue to lose weight satisfactorily.
The other way to break up a plateau is by giving a non-mercurial diuretic for one day. This is simpler for the patient but we prefer the apple-day as we sometimes find that though the diuretic is very effective on the following day it may take two to three days before the normal daily reduction is resumed, throwing the patient into a new fit of

despair. It is useless to give either an apple-day or a diuretic unless the weight has been stationary for at least four days without any dietary error having been committed.

Reaching a Former Level

The third type of interruption in the regular loss of weight may last much longer - ten days to two weeks. Fortunately, it is rare and only occurs in very advanced cases, and then hardly ever during the first course of treatment. It is seen only in those patients who during some period of their lives have maintained a certain fixed degree of obesity for ten years or more and have then at some time rapidly increased beyond that weight. When then in the course of treatment the former level is reached, it may take two weeks of no loss, in spite of HCG and diet, before further reduction is normally resumed.

Menstrual Interruption

The fourth type of interruption is the one which often occurs a few days before and during the menstrual period and in some women at the time of ovulation. It must also be mentioned that when a woman becomes pregnant during treatment - and this is by no means uncommon - she at once ceases to lose weight. An unexplained arrest of reduction has on several occasions raised our suspicion before the first period was missed. If in such cases, menstruation is delayed, we stop injecting and do a precipitation test five days later. No pregnancy test should be carried out earlier than five days after the last injection, as otherwise the HCG may give a false positive result.
Oral contraceptives may be used during treatment.

Dietary Errors

Any interruption of the normal loss of weight which does not fit perfectly into one of those categories is always due to some possibly very minor dietary error. Similarly, any gain of more than 100 grams is invariably the result of some transgression or mistake, unless it happens on or about the day of ovulation or during the three days preceding the onset of menstruation, in which case it is ignored. In all other cases the reason for the gain must be established at once.

The patient who frankly admits that he has stepped out of his regimen when told that something has gone wrong is no problem. He is always surprised at being found out, because unless he has seen this himself he will not believe that a salted almond, a couple of potato chips, a glass of tomato juice or an extra orange will bring about a definite increase in his weight on the following day.

Very often he wants to know why extra food weighing one ounce should increase his weight by six ounces. We explain this in the following way: Under the influence of HCG the blood is saturated with food and the blood volume has adapted itself so that it can only just accommodate the 500 Calories which come in from the intestinal tract in the course of the day. Any additional income, however little this may be, cannot be accommodated and the blood is therefore forced to increase its volume sufficiently to

124

hold the extra food, which it can only do in a very diluted form. Thus it is not the weight of what is eaten that plays the determining role but rather the amount of water which the body must retain to accommodate this food.

This can be illustrated by mentioning the case of salt. In order to hold one teaspoonful of salt the body requires one liter of water, as it cannot accommodate salt in any higher concentration. Thus, if a person eats one teaspoonfull of salt his weight will go up by more than two pounds as soon as this salt is absorbed from his intestine.

To this explanation many patients reply: Well, if I put on that much every time I eat a little extra, how can I hold my weight after the treatment? It must therefore be made clear that this only happens as long as they are under HCG. When treatment is over, the blood is no longer saturated and can easily accommodate extra food without having to increase its volume. Here again the professional reader will be aware that this interpretation is a simplification of an extremely intricate physiological process which actually accounts for the phenomenon.

Salt and Reducing

While we are on the subject of salt, I can take this opportunity to explain that we make no restriction in the use of salt and insist that the patients drink large quantities of water throughout the treatment. We are out to reduce abnormal fat and are not in the least interested in such illusory weight losses as can be achieved by depriving the body of salt and by desiccating it. Though we allow the free use of salt, the daily amount taken should be roughly the same, as a sudden increase will of course be followed by a corresponding increase in weight as shown by the scale. An increase in the intake of salt is one of the most common causes for an increase in weight from one day to the next. Such an increase can be ignored, provided it is accounted for. It in no way influences the regular loss of fat.

Water

Patients are usually hard to convince that the amount of water they retain has nothing to do with the amount of water they drink. When the body is forced to retain water, it will do this at all costs. If the fluid intake is insufficient to provide all the water required, the body withholds water from the kidneys and the urine becomes scanty and highly concentrated, imposing a certain strain on the kidneys. If that is insufficient, excessive water will be with-drawn from the intestinal tract, with the result that the feces become hard and dry. On the other hand if a patient drinks more than his body requires, the surplus is promptly and easily eliminated. Trying to prevent the body from retaining water by drinking less is therefore not only futile but even harmful.

Constipation

An excess of water keeps the feces soft, and that is very important in the obese, who commonly suffer from constipation and a spastic colon. While a patient is under treatment we never permit the use of any kind of laxative taken by mouth. We explain that owing to the restricted diet it is perfectly satisfactory and normal to have an evacuation of the bowel only once every three to four days and that, provided plenty of fluids are taken, this never leads to any disturbance. Only in those patients who begin to fret after four days do we allow the use of a suppository. Patients who observe this rule find that after treatment they have a perfectly normal bowel action and this delights many of them almost as much as their loss of weight.

Investigating Dietary Errors

When the reason for a slight gain in weight is not immediately evident, it is necessary to investigate further. A patient who is unaware of having committed an error or is unwilling to admit a mistake protests indignantly when told he has done something he ought not to have done. In that atmosphere no fruitful investigation can be conducted; so we calmly explain that we are not accusing him of anything but that we know for certain from our not inconsiderable experience that something has gone wrong and that we must now sit down quietly together and try and find out what it was. Once the patient realizes that it is in his own interest that he play an active and not merely a passive role in this search, the reason for the setback is almost invariably discovered. Having been through hundreds of such sessions, we are nearly always able to distinguish the deliberate liar from the patient who is merely fooling himself or is really unaware of having erred.

Liars and Fools

When we see obese patients there are generally two of us present in order to speed up routine handling. Thus when we have to investigate a rise in weight, a glance is sufficient to make sure that we agree or disagree. If after a few questions we both feel reasonably sure that the patient is deliberately lying, we tell him that this is our opinion and warn him that unless he comes clean we may refuse further treatment. The way he reacts to this furnishes additional proof whether we are on the right track or not we now very rarely make a mistake.

If the patient breaks down and confesses, we melt and are all forgiveness and treatment proceeds. Yet if such performances have to be repeated more than two or three times, we refuse further treatment. This happens in less than 1% of our cases. If the patient is stubborn and will not admit what he has been up to, we usually give him one more chance and continue treatment even though we have been unable to find the reason for his gain. In many such cases there is no repetition, and frequently the patient does then confess a few days later after he has thought things over.

The patient who is fooling himself is the one who has committed some trifling, offense against the rules but who has been able to convince himself that this is of no importance and cannot possibly account for the gain in weight. Women seem particularly prone to getting themselves entangled in such delusions. On the other hand, it does frequently happen that a patient will in the midst of a conversation unthinkingly spear an olive or forget that he has already eaten his breadstick.

A mother preparing food for the family may out of sheer habit forget that she must not taste the sauce to see whether it needs more salt. Sometimes a rich maiden aunt cannot be offended by refusing a cup of tea into which she has put two teaspoons of sugar, thoughtfully remembering the patient's taste from previous occasions. Such incidents are legion and are usually confessed without hesitation, but some patients seem genuinely able to forget these lapses and remember them with a visible shock only after insistent questioning.

In these cases we go carefully over the day. Sometimes the patient has been invited to a meal or gone to a restaurant, naively believing that the food has actually been prepared exactly according to instructions. They will say: "Yes, now that I come to think of it the steak did seem a bit bigger than the one I have at home, and it did taste better; maybe there was a little fat on it, though I specially told them to cut it all away". Sometimes the breadsticks were broken and a few fragments eaten, and "Maybe they were a little more than one". It is not uncommon for patients to place too much reliance on their memory of the diet-sheet and start eating carrots, beans or peas and then to seem genuinely surprised when their attention is called to the fact that these are forbidden, as they have not been listed.

Cosmetics

When no dietary error is elicited we turn to cosmetics. Most women find it hard to believe that fats, oils, creams and ointments applied to the skin are absorbed and interfere with weight reduction by HCG just as if they had been eaten. This almost incredible sensitivity to even such very minor increases in nutritional intake is a peculiar feature of the HCG method. For instance, we find that persons who habitually handle organic fats, such as workers in beauty parlors, masseurs, butchers, etc. never show what we consider a satisfactory loss of weight unless they can avoid fat coming into contact with their skin.

The point is so important that I will illustrate it with two cases. A lady who was cooperating perfectly suddenly increased half a pound. Careful questioning brought nothing to light. She had certainly made no dietary error nor had she used any kind of face cream, and she was already in the menopause. As we felt that we could trust her implicitly, we left the question suspended. Yet

just as she was about to leave the consulting room she suddenly stopped, turned and snapped her fingers. "I've got it," she said. This is what had happened : She had bought herself a new set of make-up pots and bottles and, using her fingers, had transferred her large assortment of cosmetics to the new containers in anticipation of the day she would be able to use them again after her treatment.

The other case concerns a man who impressed us as being very conscientious. He was about 20 lbs. overweight but did not lose satisfactorily from the onset of treatment. Again and again we tried to find the reason but with no success, until one day he said:"I never told you this, but I have a glass eye. In fact, I have a whole set of them. I frequently change them, and every time I do that I put a special ointment in my eyesocket.. Do you think that could have anything to do with it?" As we thought just that, we asked him to stop using this ointment, and from that day on his weight-loss was regular.

We are particularly averse to those modern cosmetics which contain hormones, as any interference with endocrine regulations during treatment must be absolutely avoided. Many women whose skin has in the course of years become adjusted to the use of fat containing cosmetics find that their skin gets dry as soon as they stop using them. In such cases we permit the use of plain mineral oil, which has no nutritional value. On the other hand, mineral oil should not be used in preparing the food, first because of its undesirable laxative quality, and second because it absorbs some fat-soluble vitamins, which are then lost in the stool. We do permit the use of lipstick, powder and such lotions as are entirely free of fatty substances. We also allow brilliantine to be used on the hair but it must not be rubbed into the scalp. Obviously sun-tan oil is prohibited.

Many women are horrified when told that for the duration of treatment they cannot use face creams or have facial massages. They fear that this and the loss of weight will ruin their complexion. They can be fully reassured. Under treatment normal fat is restored to the skin, which rapidly becomes fresh and turgid, making the expression much more youthful. This is a characteristic of the HCG method which is a constant source of wonder to patients who have experienced or seen in others the facial ravages produced by the usual methods of reducing. An obese woman of 70 obviously cannot expect to have her pued face reduced to normal without a wrinkle, but it is remarkable how youthful her face remains in spite of her age.

The Voice

Incidentally, another interesting feature of the HCG method is that it does not ruin a singing voice. The typically obese prima donna usually finds that when she tries to reduce, the timbre of her voice is liable to change, and understandably this terrifies her. Under HCG this does not happen; indeed, in many cases the voice improves and the breathing invariably does. We have had many cases of professional singers very carefully controlled by expert voice teachers, and the maestros have been so enthusiastic that they now frequently send us patients.

Other Reasons for a Gain

Apart from diet and cosmetics there can be a few other reasons for a small rise in weight. Some patients unwittingly take chewing gum, throat pastilles, vitamin pills, cough syrups etc., without realizing that the sugar or fats they contain may interfere with a regular loss of weight. Sex hormones or cortisone in its various modern forms must be avoided, though oral contraceptives are permitted. In fact the only self-medication we allow is aspirin for a headache, though headaches almost invariably disappear after a week of treatment, particularly if of the migraine type.

Occasionally we allow a sleeping tablet or a tranquilizer, but patients should be told that while under treatment they need and may get less sleep. For instance, here in Italy where it is customary to sleep during the siesta which lasts from one to four in the afternoon most patients find that though they lie down they are unable to sleep.

We encourage swimming and sun bathing during treatment, but it should be remembered that a severe sunburn always produces a temporary rise in weight, evidently due to water retention. The same may be seen when a patient gets a common cold during treatment. Finally, the weight can temporarily increase paradoxical though this may sound - after an exceptional physical exertion of long duration leading to a feeling of exhaustion. A game of tennis, a vigorous swim, a run, a ride on horseback or a round of golf do not have this effect; but a long trek, a day of skiing, rowing or cycling or dancing into the small hours usually result in a gain of weight on the following day, unless the patient is in perfect training. In patients coming from abroad, where they always use their cars, we often see this effect after a strenuous day of shopping on foot, sightseeing and visits to galleries and museums. Though the extra muscular effort involved does consume some additional Calories, this appears to be offset by the retention of water which the tired circulation cannot at once eliminate.

Appetite-reducing Drugs

We hardly ever use amphetamines, the appetite-reducing drugs such as Dexedrin, Dexamil, Preludin, etc., as there seems to be no need for them during the HCG treatment. The only time we find them useful is when a patient is, for impelling and unforeseen reasons, obliged to forego the injections for three to four days and yet wishes to continue the diet so that he need not interrupt the course.

Unforeseen Interruptions of Treatment

If an interruption of treatment lasting more than four days is necessary, the patient must increase his diet to at least 800 Calories by adding meat, eggs, cheese, and milk to his diet after the third day, as otherwise he will find himself so hungry and weak that he is unable to go about his usual occupation. If the interval lasts less than two weeks the patient can directly resume injections and the 500-Calorie diet, but if the interruption lasts longer he must again eat normally until he has had his third injection.

When a patient knows beforehand that he will have to travel and be absent for more than four days, it is always better to stop injections three days before he is due to leave so that he can have the three days of strict dieting which are necessary after the last injection at home. This saves him from the almost impossible task of having to arrange the 500 Calorie diet while en route, and he can thus enjoy a much greater dietary freedom from the day of his departure. Interruptions occurring before 20 effective injections have been given are most undesirable, because with less than that number of injections some weight is liable to be regained. After the 20th injection an unavoidable interruption is merely a loss of time.

Muscular Fatigue

Towards the end of a full course, when a good deal of fat has been rapidly lost, some patients complain that lifting a weight or climbing stairs requires a greater muscular effort than before. They feel neither breathlessness nor exhaustion but simply that their muscles have to work harder. This phenomenon, which disappears soon after the end of the treatment, is caused by the removal of abnormal fat deposited between, in, and around the muscles. The removal of this fat makes the muscles too long, and so in order to achieve a certain skeletal movement - say the bending of an arm - the muscles have to perform greater contraction than before. Within a short while the muscle adjusts itself perfectly to the new situation, but under HCG the loss of fat is so rapid that this adjustment cannot keep up with it. Patients often have to be reassured that this does not mean that they are "getting weak". This phenomenon does not occur in patients who regularly take vigorous exercise and continue to do so during treatment.

Massage

I never allow any kind of massage during treatment. It is entirely unnecessary and merely disturbs a very delicate process which is going on in the tissues. Few indeed are the masseurs and masseuses who can resist the temptation to knead and hammer abnormal fat deposits. In the course of rapid reduction it is sometimes possible to pick up a fold of skin which has not yet had time to adjust itself, as it always does under HCG, to the changed figure. This fold contains its normal subcutaneous fat and may be almost an inch thick. It is one of the main objects of the HCG treatment to keep that fat there. Patients and their masseurs do not always understand this and give this fat a working-over. I have seen such patients who were as black and blue as if they had received a sound thrashing.

In my opinion, massage, thumping, rolling, kneading, and shivering undertaken for the purpose of reducing abnormal fat can do nothing but harm. We once had the honor of treating the proprietress of a high class institution that specialized in such antics. She had the audacity to confess that she was taking our treatment to convince her clients of the efficacy of her methods, which she had found useless in her own case.

How anyone in his right mind is able to believe that fatty tissue can be shifted mechanically or be made to vanish by squeezing is beyond my comprehension. The only effect obtained is severe bruising. The torn tissue then forms scars, and these slowly contract making the fatty tissue even harder and more unyielding.

A lady once consulted us for her most ungainly legs. Large masses of fat bulged over the ankles of her tiny feet, and there were about 40 lbs. too much on her hips and thighs. We assured her that this overweight could be lost and that her ankles would markedly improve in the process. Her treatment progressed most satisfactorily but to our surprise there was no improvement in her ankles. We then discovered that she had for years been taking every kind of mechanical, electric and heat treatment for her legs and that she had made up her mind to resort to plastic surgery if we failed.

Re-examining the fat above her ankles, we found that it was unusually hard. We attributed this to the countless minor injuries inflicted by kneading. These injuries had healed but had left a tough network of connective scar-tissue in which the fat was imprisoned. Ready to try anything, she was put to bed for the remaining three weeks of her first course with her lower legs tightly strapped in unyielding bandages. Every day the pressure was increased. The combination of HCG, diet and strapping brought about a marked improvement in the shape of her ankles. At the end of her first course she returned to her home abroad. Three months later she came back for her second course. She had maintained both her weight and the improvement of her ankles. The same procedure was repeated, and after five weeks she left the hospital with a normal weight and legs that, if not exactly shapely, were at least unobtrusive. Where no such injuries of the tissues have been inflicted by inappropriate methods of treatment, these drastic measures are never necessary.

Blood Sugar

Towards the end of a course or when a patient has nearly reached his normal weight it occasionally happens that the blood sugar drops below normal, and we have even seen this in patients who had an abnormally high blood sugar before treatment. Such an attack of hypoglycemia is almost identical with the one seen in diabetics who have taken too much insulin. The attack comes on suddenly; there is the same feeling of light-headedness, weakness in the knees, trembling, and unmotivated sweating; but under HCG, hypoglycemia does not produce any feeling of hunger. All these symptoms are almost instantly relieved by taking two heaped teaspoons of sugar.

In the course of treatment the possibility of such an attack is explained to those patients who are in a phase in which a drop in blood sugar may occur. They are instructed to keep sugar or glucose sweets handy, particularly when driving a car. They are also told to watch the effect of taking sugar very carefully and report the following day. This is important, because anxious patients to whom such an attack has been explained are apt to take sugar unnecessarily, in which case it inevitably produces a gain in weight and does not dramatically relieve the symptoms for which it was taken, proving that these were not due to hypoglycemia. Some patients mistake the effects of emotional stress for hypoglycemia. When the symptoms are quickly relieved by sugar this is proof that they were indeed due to an abnormal lowering of the blood sugar, and in that case there is no increase in the weight on the following day. We always suggest that sugar be taken if the patient is in doubt.

Once such an attack has been relieved with sugar we have never seen it recur on the immediately subsequent days, and only very rarely does a patient have two such attacks separated by several days during a course of treatment. In patients who have not eaten sufficiently during the first two days of treatment we sometimes give sugar when the minor symptoms usually felt during the first three days of treatment continue beyond that time, and in some cases this has seemed to speed up the euphoria ordinarily associated with the HCG method.

The Ratio of Pounds to Inches

An interesting feature of the HCG method is that, regardless of how fat a patient is, the greatest circumference -- abdomen or hips as the case may be is reduced at a constant rate which is extraordinarily close to 1 cm. per kilogram of weight lost. At the beginning of treatment the change in measurements is somewhat greater than this, but at the end of a course it is almost invariably found that the girth is as many centimeters less as the number of kilograms by which the weight has been reduced. I have never seen this clear cut relationship in patients that try to reduce by dieting only.

Preparing the Solution

Human chorionic gonadotrophin comes on the market as a highly soluble powder which is the pure substance extracted from the urine of pregnant women. Such preparations are carefully standardized, and any brand made by a reliable pharmaceutical company is probably as good as any other. The substance should be extracted from the urine and not from the placenta, and it must of course be of human and not of animal origin. The powder is sealed in ampoules or in rubber-capped bottles in varying amounts which are stated in International Units. In this form HCG is stable; however, only such preparations should be used that have the date of manufacture and the date of expiry clearly stated on the label or package. A suitable solvent is always supplied in a separate ampoule in the same package.

Once HCG is in solution it is far less stable. It may be kept at room-temperature for two to three days, but if the solution must be kept longer it should always be refrigerated. When treating only one or two cases simultaneously, vials containing a small number of units say 1000 I.U. should be used. The 10 cc. of solvent which is supplied by the manufacturer is injected into the rubber- capped bottle containing the HCG, and the powder must dissolve instantly. Of this solution 1.25 cc. are withdrawn for each injection. One such bottle of 1000 I.U. therefore furnishes 8 injections. When more than one patient is being treated, they should not each have their own bottle but rather all be injected from the same vial and a fresh solution made when this is empty.

As we are usually treating a fair number of patients at the same time, we prefer to use vials containing 5000 units. With these the manufactures also supply 10 cc. of solvent. Of such a solution 0.25 cc. contain the 125 I.U., which is the standard dose for all cases and which should never be exceeded. This small amount is awkward to handle accurately (it requires an insulin syringe) and is wasteful, because there is a loss of solution in the nozzle of the syringe and in the needle. We therefore prefer a higher dilution, which we prepare in the following way: The solvent supplied is injected into the rubbercapped bottle containing the 5000 I.U . As these bottles are too small to hold more solvent, we withdraw 5 cc., inject it into an empty rubber-capped bottle and add 5 cc. of normal saline to each bottle. This gives us 10 cc. of solution in each bottle, and of this solution 0.5 cc. contains 125 I.U. This amount is convenient to inject with an ordinary syringe.

Injecting

HCG produces little or no tissue-reaction, it is completely painless and in the many thousands of injections we have given we have never seen an inflammatory or suppurative reaction at the site of the injection.

One should avoid leaving a vacuum in the bottle after preparing the solution or after withdrawal of the amount required for the injections as otherwise alcohol used for sterilizing a frequently perforated rubber cap might be drawn into the solution. When sharp needles are used, it sometimes happens that a little bit of rubber is punched out of the rubber cap and can be seen as a small black speck floating in the solution. As these bits of rubber are heavier than the solution they rapidly settle out, and it is thus easy to avoid drawing them into the syringe.

We use very fine needles that are two inches long and inject deep intragluteally in the outer upper quadrant of the buttocks. The injection should if possible not be given into the superficial fat layers, which in very obese patients must be compressed so as to enable the needle to reach the muscle. Obviously needles and syringes must be carefully washed, sterilized and handled aseptically. It is also important that the daily injection should be given at intervals as close to 24 hours as possible. Any attempt to economize in time by giving larger doses at longer intervals is doomed to produce less satisfactory results.

There are hardly any contraindications to the HCG method. Treatment can be continued in the presence of abscesses, suppuration, large infected wounds and major fractures. Surgery and general anesthesia are no reason to stop and we have given treatment during a severe attack of malaria. Acne or boils are no contraindication; the former usually clears up, and furunculosis comes to an end. Thrombophlebitis is no contraindication, and we have treated several obese patients with HCG and the 500-Calorie diet while suffering from this condition. Our impression has been that in obese patients the phlebitis does rather better and certainly no worse than under the usual treatment alone. This also applies to patients suffering from varicose ulcers which tend to heal rapidly.

Fibroids
While uterine fibroids seem to be in no way affected by HCG in the doses we use, we have found that very large, externally palpable uterine myomas are apt to give trouble. We are convinced that this is entirely due to the rather sudden disappearance of fat from the pelvic bed upon which they rest and that it is the weight of the tumor pressing on the underlying tissues which accounts for the discomfort or pain which may arise during treatment. While we disregard even fair-sized or multiple myomas, we insist that very large ones be operated before treatment. We have had patients present themselves for reducing fat from their abdomen who showed no signs of obesity, but had a large abdominal tumor.

Gallstones

Small stones in the gall bladder may in patients who have recently had typical colics cause more frequent colics under treatment with HCG. This may be due to the almost complete absence of fat from the diet, which prevents the normal emptying of the gall bladder. Before undertaking treatment we explain to such patients that there is a risk of more frequent and possibly severe symptoms and that it may become necessary to operate. If they are prepared to take this risk and provided they agree to undergo an operation if we consider this imperative, we proceed with treatment, as after weight reduction with HCG the operative risk is considerably reduced in an obese patient. In such cases we always give a drug which stimulates the flow of bile, and in the majority of cases nothing untoward happens. On the other hand, we have looked for and not found any evidence to suggest that the HCG treatment leads to the formation of gallstones as pregnancy sometimes does.

The Heart

Disorders of the heart are not as a rule contraindications. In fact, the removal of abnormal fat - particularly from the heart-muscle and from the surrounding of the coronary arteries - can only be beneficial in cases of myocardial weakness, and many such patients are referred to us by cardiologists. Within the first week of treatment all patients - not only heart cases - remark that they have lost much of their breathlessness.

Coronary Occlusion

In obese patients who have recently survived a coronary occlusion, we adopt the following procedure in collaboration with the cardiologist. We wait until no further electrocardiographic changes have occurred for a period of three months. Routine treatment is then started under careful control and it is usual to find a further electrocardiographic improvement of a condition which was previously stationary.

In the thousands of cases we have treated we have not once seen any sort of coronary incident occur during or shortly after treatment. The same applies to cerebral vascular accidents. Nor have we ever seen a case of thrombosis of any sort develop during treatment, even though a high blood pressure is rapidly lowered. In this respect, too, the HCG treatment resembles pregnancy.

Teeth and Vitamins

Patients whose teeth are in poor repair sometimes get more trouble under prolonged treatment, just as may occur in pregnancy. In such cases we do allow calcium and vitamin D, though not in an oily solution. The only other vitamin we permit is vitamin C, which we use in large doses combined with an antihistamine at the onset of a common cold. There is no objection to the use of an antibiotic if this is required, for instance by the dentist. In cases of bronchial asthma and hay fever we have occasionally resorted to cortisone during treatment and find that triamcinolone is the least likely to interfere with the loss of weight, but many asthmatics improve with HCG alone.

Alcohol

Obese heavy drinkers, even those bordering on alcoholism, often do surprisingly well under HCG and it is exceptional for them to take a drink while under treatment. When they do, they find that a relatively small quantity of alcohol produces intoxication. Such patients say that they do not feel the need to drink. This may in part be due to the euphoria which the treatment produces and in part to the complete absence of the need for quick sustenance from which most obese patients suffer.

Though we have had a few cases that have continued abstinence long after treatment, others relapse as soon as they are back on a normal diet. We have a few "regular customers" who, having once been reduced to their normal weight, start to drink again though watching their weight. Then after some months they purposely overeat in order to gain sufficient weight for another course of HCG which temporarily gets them out of their drinking routine. We do not particularly welcome such cases, but we see no reason for refusing their request.

Tuberculosis

It is interesting that obese patients suffering from inactive pulmonary tuberculosis can be safely treated. We have under very careful control treated patients as early as three months after they were pronounced inactive and have never seen a relapse occur during or shortly after treatment. In fact, we only have one case on our records in which active tuberculosis developed in a young man about one year after a treatment which had lasted three weeks. Earlier X-rays showed a calcified spot from a childhood infection which had not produced clinical symptoms. There was a family history of tuberculosis, and his illness started under adverse conditions which certainly had nothing to do with the treatment. Residual calcifications from an early infection are exceedingly common, and we never consider them a contraindication to treatment.

The Painful Heel

In obese patients who have been trying desperately to keep their weight down by severe dieting, a curious symptom sometimes occurs. They complain of an unbearable pain in their heels which they feel only while standing or walking. As soon as they take the weight off their heels the pain ceases. These cases are the bane of the rheumatologists and orthopedic surgeons who have treated them before they come to us. All the usual investigations are entirely negative, and there is not the slightest response to anti-rheumatic medication or physiotherapy. The pain may be so severe that the patients are obliged to give up their occupation, and they are not infrequently labeled as a case of hysteria. When their heels are carefully examined one finds that the sole is softer than normal and that the heel bone - the calcaneus - can be distinctly felt, which is not the case in a normal foot.

We interpret the condition as a lack of the hard fatty pad on which the calcaneus rests and which protects both the bone and the skin of the sole from pressure. This fat is like a springy cushion which carries the weight of the body. Standing on a heel in which this fat is missing or reduced must obviously be very painful. In their efforts to keep their weight down these patients have consumed this normal structural fat.

Those patients who have a normal or subnormal weight while showing the typically obese fat deposits are made to eat to capacity, often much against their will, for one week. They gain weight rapidly but there is no improvement in the painful heels. They are then started on the routine HCG treatment. Overweight patients are treated immediately. In both cases the pain completely disappears in 10-20 days of dieting, usually around the 15th day of treatment, and so far no case has had a relapse though we have been able to follow up such patients for years.

We are particularly interested in these cases, as they furnish further proof of the contention that HCG + 500 Calories not only removes abnormal fat but actually permits normal fat to be replaced, in spite of the deficient food intake. It is certainly not so that the mere loss of weight reduces the pain, because it frequently disappears before the weight the patient had prior to the period of forced feeding is reached.

The Skeptical Patient

Any doctor who starts using the HCG method for the first time will have considerable difficulty, particularly if he himself is not fully convinced, in making patients believe that they will not feel hungry on 500 Calories and that their face will not collapse. New patients always anticipate the phenomena they know so well from previous treatments and diets and are incredulous when told that these will not occur. We overcome all this by letting new patients spend a little time in the waiting room with older hands, who can always be relied upon to allay these fears with evangelistic zeal, often demonstrating the finer points on their own body.

A waiting-room filled with obese patients who congregate daily is a sort of group therapy. They compare notes and pop back into the waiting room after the consultation to announce the score of the last 24 hours to an enthralled audience. They cross-check on their diets and sometimes confess sins which they try to hide from us, usually with the result that the patient in whom they have confided palpitatingly tattles the whole disgraceful story to us with a "But don't let her know I told you."

Concluding a Course

When the three days of dieting after the last injection are over, the patients are told that they may now eat anything they please, except sugar and starch provided they faithfully observe one simple rule. This rule is that they must have their own portable bathroom-scale always at hand, particularly while traveling. They must without fail weigh themselves every morning as they get out of bed, having first emptied their bladder. If they are in the habit of having breakfast in bed, they must weigh before breakfast.

It takes about 3 weeks before the weight reached at the end of the treatment becomes stable, i.e. does not show violent fluctuations after an occasional excess. During this period patients must realize that the so-called carbohydrates, that is sugar, rice, bread, potatoes, pastries, etc, are by far the most dangerous. If no carbohydrates whatsoever are eaten, fats can be indulged in somewhat more liberally and even small quantities of alcohol, such as a glass of wine with meals, does no harm, but as soon as fats and starch are combined things are very liable to get out of hand. This has to be observed very carefully during the first 3 weeks after the treatment is ended otherwise disappointments are almost sure to occur.

Skipping a Meal

As long as their weight stays within two pounds of the weight reached on the day of the last injection, patients should take no notice of any increase but the moment the scale goes beyond two pounds, even if this is only a few ounces, they must on that same day entirely skip breakfast and lunch but take plenty to drink. In the evening they must eat a huge steak with only an apple or a raw tomato. Of course this rule applies only to the morning weight. Ex-obese patients should never check their weight during the day, as there may be wide fluctuations and these are merely alarming and confusing.

It is of utmost importance that the meal is skipped on the same day as the scale registers an increase of more than two pounds and that missing the meals is not postponed until the following day. If a meal is skipped on the day in which a gain is registered in the morning this brings about an immediate drop of often over a pound. But if the skipping of the meal - and skipping means literally skipping, not just having a light meal - is postponed the phenomenon does not occur and several days of strict dieting may be necessary to correct the situation.

Most patients hardly ever need to skip a meal. If they have eaten a heavy lunch they feel no desire to eat their dinner, and in this case no increase takes place. If they keep their weight at the point reached at the end of the treatment, even a heavy dinner does not bring about an increase of two pounds on the next morning and does not therefore call for any special measures. Most patients are surprised how small their appetite has become and yet how much they can eat without gaining weight. They no longer suffer from an abnormal appetite and feel satisfied with much less food than before. In fact, they are usually disappointed that they cannot manage their first normal meal, which they have been planning for weeks.

Losing more Weight

An ex-patient should never gain more than two pounds without immediately correcting this, but it is equally undesirable that more than two lbs. be lost after treatment, because a greater loss is always achieved at the expense of normal fat. Any normal fat that is lost is invariably regained as soon as more food is taken, and it often happens that this rebound overshoots the upper two lbs. limit.

Trouble After Treatment

Two difficulties may be encountered in the immediate post-treatment period. When a patient has consumed all his abnormal fat or, when after a full course, the injection has temporarily lost its efficacy owing to the body having gradually evolved a counter regulation, the patient at once begins to feel much more hungry and even weak. In spite of repeated warnings, some over-enthusiastic patients do not report this. However, in about two days the fact that they are being undernourished becomes visible in their faces, and treatment is then stopped at once. In such cases - and only in such cases - we allow a very slight increase in the diet, such as an extra apple, 150 grams of meat or two or three extra breadsticks during the three days of dieting after the last injection.

When abnormal fat is no longer being put into circulation either because it has been consumed or because immunity has set in, this is always felt by the patient as sudden, intolerable and constant hunger. In this sense, the HCG method is completely self-limiting. With HCG it is impossible to reduce a patient, however enthusiastic, beyond his normal weight. As soon as no more abnormal fat is being issued, the body starts consuming normal fat, and this is always regained as soon as ordinary feeding is resumed. The patient then finds that the 2-3 lbs. he has lost during the last days of treatment are immediately regained. A meal is skipped and maybe a pound is lost. The next day this pound is regained, in spite of a careful watch over the food intake. In a few days a tearful patient is back in the consulting room, convinced that her case is a failure.

All that is happening is that the essential fat lost at the end of the treatment, owing to the patient's reluctance to report a much greater hunger, is being replaced. The weight at which such a patient must stabilize thus lies 2-3 lbs. higher than the weight reached at the end of the treatment. Once this higher basic level is established, further difficulties in controlling the weight at the new point of stabilization hardly arise.

Beware of Over-enthusiasm

The other trouble which is frequently encountered immediately after treatment is again due to over-enthusiasm. Some patients cannot believe that they can eat fairly normally without regaining weight. They disregard the advice to eat anything they please except sugar and starch and want to play safe. They try more or less to continue the 500-Calorie diet on which they felt so well during treatment and make only minor variations, such as replacing the meat with an egg, cheese, or a glass of milk. To their horror they find that in spite of this bravura, their weight goes up. So, following instructions, they skip one meager lunch and at night eat only a little salad and drink a pot of unsweetened tea, becoming increasingly hungry and weak. The next morning they find that they have increased yet another pound. They feel terrible, and even the dreaded swelling of their ankles is back. Normally we check our patients one week after they have been eating freely, but these cases return in a few days. Either their eyes are filled with tears or they angrily imply that when we told them to eat normally we were just fooling them.

Protein deficiency

Here too, the explanation is quite simple. During treatment the patient has been only just above the verge of protein deficiency and has had the advantage of protein being fed back into his system from the breakdown of fatty tissue. Once the treatment is over there is no more HCG in the body and this process no longer takes place. Unless an adequate amount of protein is eaten as soon as the treatment is over, protein deficiency is bound to develop, and this inevitably causes the marked retention of water known as hunger- edema.

The treatment is very simple. The patient is told to eat two eggs for breakfast and a huge steak for lunch and dinner followed by a large helping of cheese and to phone through the weight the next morning. When these instructions are followed a stunned voice is heard to report that two lbs. have vanished overnight, that the ankles are normal but that sleep was disturbed, owing to an extraordinary need to pass large quantities of water. The patient having learned this lesson usually has no further trouble.

Relapses

As a general rule one can say that 60%-70% of our cases experience little or no difficulty in holding their weight permanently. Relapses may be due to negligence in the basic rule of daily weighing. Many patients think that this is unnecessary and that they can judge any increase from the fit of their clothes. Some do not carry their scale with them on a journey as it is cumbersome and takes a big bite out of their luggage-allowance when flying. This is a disastrous mistake, because after a course of HCG as much as 10 lbs. can be regained without any noticeable change in the fit of the clothes. The reason for this is that after treatment newly acquired fat is at first evenly distributed and does not show the former preference for certain parts of the body.

Pregnancy or the menopause may annul the effect of a previous treatment. Women who take treatment during the one year after the last menstruation - that is at the onset of the menopause - do just as well as others, but among them the relapse rate is higher until the menopause is fully established. The period of one year after the last menstruation applies only to women who are not being treated with ovarian hormones. If these are taken, the premenopausal period may be indefinitely prolonged.

Late teenage girls who suffer from attacks of compulsive eating have by far the worst record of all as far as relapses are concerned.

Patients who have once taken the treatment never seem to hesitate to come back for another short course as soon as they notice that their weight is once again getting out of hand. They come quite cheerfully and hopefully, assured that they can be helped again. Repeat courses are often even more satisfactory than the first treatment and have the advantage, as do second courses, that the patient already, knows that he will feel comfortable throughout.
Plan of a Normal Course

125 I.U. of HCG daily (except during menstruation) until 40 injections have been given.

Until 3rd injection forced feeding.

After 3rd injection, 500 Calorie diet to be continued until 72 hours after the last injection.

For the following 3 weeks, all foods allowed except starch and sugar in any form (careful with very sweet fruit).

After 3 weeks, very gradually add starch in small quantities, always controlled by morning weighing.

CONCLUSION

The HCG + diet method can bring relief to every case of obesity, but the method is not simple. It is very time consuming and requires perfect cooperation between physician and patient. Each case must be handled individually, and the physician must have time to answer questions, allay fears and remove misunderstandings. He must also check the patient daily. When something goes wrong he must at once investigate until he finds the reason for any gain that may have occurred. In most cases it is useless to hand the patient a diet-sheet and let the nurse give him a "shot."

The method involves a highly complex bodily mechanism, and even though our theory may be wrong the physician must make himself some sort of picture of what is actually happening; otherwise he will not be able to deal with such difficulties as may arise during treatment.

I must beg those trying the method for the first time to adhere very strictly to the technique and the interpretations here outlined and thus treat a few hundred cases before embarking on experiments of their own, and until then refrain from introducing innovations, however thrilling they may seem. In a new method, innovations or departures from the original technique can only be usefully evaluated against a substantial background of experience with what is at the moment the orthodox procedure. I have tried to cover all the problems that come to my mind. Yet a bewildering array of new questions keeps arising, and my interpretations are still fluid. In particular, I have never had an opportunity of conducting the laboratory investigations which are so necessary for a theoretical understanding of clinical observations, and I can only hope that those more fortunately placed will in time be able to fill this gap.

The problems of obesity are perhaps not so dramatic as the problems of cancer, or polio, but they often cause life long suffering. How many promising careers have been ruined by excessive fat; how many lives have been shortened. If some way -however cumbersome - can be found to cope effectively with this universal problem of modern civilized man, our world will be a happier place for countless fellow men and women.

******** I have left the Glossary and the Literary References to the Use of Chorionic GonadotrophinIn Obesity
out of this book in order to save space. You may find it online if you
wish.*************

POUNDS AND INCHES Privately printed: obtainable only from A.T.W. Simeons, Salvator Mundi International Hospital, Rome, Italy
E.P. Dutton, New York (hardback) Dutton Paperbacks, New York